100
LIFE or
DEATH
FOODS

A Scientific Guide to Foods That Prolong Life or Kill You Prematurely

Jean Carper
1 New York Times Best-Selling Author

Copyright 2024 by Jean Carper

All rights reserved under the International and
Pan-American Copyright Conventions.
Printed in the United States of America

No part of this publication may be reproduced,
distributed, stored in a retrieval system, or transmitted in
any form or by any means, electronic, or otherwise,
without the prior written permission of the copyright
holder.

Jean Carper,
1500 Von Phister Street,
Key West, Florida 33040

First Edition: December 2023

NON-FICTION / Health & Fitness > Diseases

ISBN:979-887-08054-2-9, Trade Paper
Copyright © 2023, Jean Carper
Electronic compilation/ paperback edition
copyright © 2023 By Jean Carper

To Three Incredible Women:

Natella Carper, my mother who lived to be 96,
Lola Boyer, her mother who lived to be 82 and
Lozana Peters, her mother who lived to be 89.

OTHER BOOKS BY JEAN CARPER

100 Simple Things You Can Do to Prevent Alzheimer's

Food Your Miracle Medicine

The Food Pharmacy

Miracle Cures

Stop Aging Now!

Your Miracle Brain

The Miracle Heart

Health Care USA

Jean Carper's Total Nutrition Guide

Jean Carper's Complete Healthy Cookbook

Eating May Be Hazardous to Your Health

CONTENTS

Introduction: *Add Ten Years to Your Lifespan*

How Specific Foods, Drinks, Diets, & Other Food Factors Affect Longevity

Apple: *Adds One Third to Life Expectancy*
Avocado: *Boosts Heart Functioning*
Banana: *Discourages Cancer*
Beans & Legumes: *Universal Champions of Life*
Beer: *Dilutes Life Expectancy*
Beet: *Revs Up Brain Energy*
Berries: *Amazing Defenders Against Death*
Beverages with Alcohol: *Unsafe Sip by Sip*
Blue Zones Diet: *Ideal for Centenarians*
Bread: *White is Death's Best Friend*
Breakfast: *Skipping Brings Death Sooner*
Butter & Margarine: *Longevity Detractors*
Cabbage*: Spectacular Life Preserver*
Caffeine: *Keeps You Awake and Alive!*
Calories: *Overloads Destroy Longevity*

vii

Candy: *Death's Faithful Accomplice*
Carbohydrates: *They Mess with Mortality*
Carrot: *Formidable Foe of Cancer*
Celery: *Mimic the Man with a Juicer*
Cereal: *Choose Lifesavers Not Killers*
Cheese: *Not Likely the Kiss of Death*
Chili Peppers: *Red Hot Life Extenders*
Chocolate: *Super-Food with a Dark Side*
Coffee: *Sure Bet to Boost Longevity*
Corn: *Old World Pro-Life Staple*
Cruciferous Vegetables: *Totems for Long Life*
Dash Diet: *Famous Blood Pressure Downer*
Diet Sodas: *They Kill You, Too, But Faster*
Dietary Patterns: *Best and Worst Diets*
Eating Disorders: *Skyrocketing Deaths*
Eggs: *The Scare Factor is Back*
Eggplant: *Ancient Staple with Purple Power*
Fasting: *Controversial Way to Prolong Life*
Fats & Oils: *The Best, Worse, and Just Awful*
Fermented Food: *"Bad" Food for Longer Life*
Fiber: *King of Longevity*
Fish: *First Course for Aspiring Immortals*
Flavonoids: *Life-Stretching Antioxidants*
Fried Foods: *Everybody's Fatal Attraction*
Fruits & Vegetables: *Longevity Super Stars*
Garlic: *The Grandee of Lifesaving Herbs*
Glycemic Rating: *Major Clue to Longevity*

Grapes & Raisins: *Resveratrol Slows Aging*
Green Leafy Veggies: *Essential for Longevity*
Herbs & Spices: *Tiny Doses Extend Survival*
Honey & Maple Syrup: *Super Sugar Busters*
Ice Cream: *Cool Way to Flirt with Death*
Japanese Diet: *Adds Years to Your Earth Time*
Juices: *Not the Superfood You Think*
Kale: *God's Gift to Longevity*
Keto Diet: *Controversial and Risky*
Meat, Cured: *Bacon, Ham, Hot Dogs, etc.*
 Ferocious Carcinogens
Meat, Uncured: *Beef, Lamb, Pork, Veal*
 Powerful Assassins
Mediterranean Diet: *World-Famous Diet*
Mediterranean Green Diet: *Beyond Classic*
Milk: *How Much is Harmful?*
Mind Diet: *Puts Death on Dramatic Hold*
Mushroom: *Behold the "Longevity Vitamin"*
Nuts: *Astonishing Morsels of Longevity*
Oats: *Superstar for All Time*
Obesity: *The Truth About Death and Fat*
Olives & Oil: *Best Oil for a Long Life*
Onion: *A Star but Not Quite a Superstar*
Pomegranate: *Prehistoric Miracle Fruit*
Potato: *Fried Foods from Hell*
Poultry & White Meat: *Better Than Dark*
Protein: *Plant or Animal, Deadly Difference*

Rice: *Go for Brown, Not White*
Salt & Sodium: *Thieves of Longevity*
Saturated Fats: *Not the Killers You Imagine*
Seaweed: *Can a Million Japanese Be Wrong?*
Shellfish: *Untrustworthy Sea Fare*
Soybeans: *Say Yes to Tofu, Miso, Edamame*
Sugar: *Imposes a Hefty Death Tax*
Sugary Beverages: *Killers On the Loose*
Sweet Potato: *Perfect for Centenarians*
Tea: *Dispensing Longevity for 40 Centuries*
Telomere-Factor: *New Secret to Immortality*
Tomato: *Packed with Lifegiving Antioxidants*
Triglycerides: *Death Threats to the Heart*
Ultra-Processed Foods: *They Kill You Young*
Vegetarian Diet: *Powerful Longevity Secrets*
Vinegar: *Extends Life by the Spoonful*
Vitamin Supplements: *Death Cares Little*
Western Diet: *Blueprint for Premature Death*
Whole Grains: *Absolute Must for a Long Life*
Wine: *A Glass or Not?*
Yogurt: *Gives Women a Longer Life*
Appendix Bibliography
About the Author

Introduction

Add Ten Years to Your Lifespan

Every bit of food you eat releases an explosion of active pharmacological chemicals that circulate in your body, infusing life or death, creating or destroying cells, preventing or fostering disease and accurately predicting whether you will have a long life or early demise.

Food is not neutral. It is not a biological deaf mute, impassive, or inert. It is a potent missile of health or malice, relentlessly firing its secret chemical weapons into your blood, bones, muscles, tissues, and skin.

In 1988 I authored a pioneering book, *The Food Pharmacy*, exploring the bold new idea that food is a complex drug with multiple powers to influence disease, death, and longevity.

More than three decades later, a flood of new research verifies that what you eat definitively slows or accelerates aging and shortens or lengthens your life. The massive details of this amazing, but largely unknown and overwhelming research are available in the National Library of Medicine, at the National Institutes of Health in Bethesda, Maryland and on other scientific databases, typically affiliated with leading universities and medical centers around the world.

I have distilled this latest research to create a unique up to date, one-stop guide to more than 100 common foods, beverages, and popular diets, revealing whether they prolong health and life or accelerate aging and death.

Virtually all foods and beverages possess a multitude of Jekyll and Hyde characteristics that affect your rate of aging and the speed of your individual march toward death. Early nutritional researchers concentrated on the impact of specific foods and food constituents on chronic diseases, such as cancer, cardiovascular disease, diabetes, kidney and lung diseases, and dementia.

Today's leading scientists increasingly focus on identifying which foods encourage longevity or premature death. Eating particular foods and beverages expands or shrinks your longevity by minutes, hours, days, weeks, months, and years. The awesome fact is science can now reveal which foods and dietary patterns are most likely to extend or shorten your life.

For the first time you will discover in this book specific foods to eat or avoid to maximize your time on earth. The latest information comes from leading investigators worldwide and is typically available through the National Institutes of Health's extensive website. A current search of the NIH database, also known as pub med, identifies 1,300,903 research articles on the impact of various foods, nutrients, and dietary patterns on life-expectancy over the last thirty-five years. This book on "life and death foods" condenses and summarizes that research.

How Long Will You Live?

Since the dawn of mankind, our average life expectancy has grown dramatically. Two and a half million years ago during the Stone Age the eldest generation was made up of teenagers. Ancient Romans and Greeks were lucky to survive into their early twenties. In the Middle Ages British royalty typically lived into their mid-forties. Between 1800 and 2000, global life expectancy, propelled by the industrial revolution, rose to age 67 and is currently 73.16 years.

Overall life expectancy in the United States peaked at 78.9 years in 2014, and then fell, partly due to the covid epidemic. In 2023 life expectancy among Americans was 74.12 for men and 79.78 for women. By 2050, the Census Bureau predicts, it will rise to 80.9 for American males and 85.3 for American females.

Expert estimates put our maximum human life expectancy at 125 years.

By no means are Americans at the top of the global heap for longevity. In 2023 the US ranked 46th in life expectancy among 193 countries. Forty-five countries with higher life expectancies than the United States include Japan, Switzerland, Italy, Spain, Australia, Sweden, France, Canada, Greece, Portugal, Germany, United Kingdom, Puerto Rico and Denmark.

Your Diet Predicts Your Longevity

Inarguably, what you eat extends or shortens your life, and the earlier you embrace life-extending foods the longer you are apt to survive. Of course, many factors besides diet influence life expectancy, including gender, genetics, hygiene, exercise, lifestyle, smoking, alcohol abuse, and physical inactivity. But your food choices are most critical in prolonging life at any age.

It is shocking to realize that "suboptimal diets" cause an estimated eleven million premature deaths yearly in what is largely a preventable global tragedy. The evidence is stunningly clear that people who eat "optimal" diets can slow their aging process and add countless years to their lives. For example, a 2022 landmark international study concluded that American women who at age 20 switch from a typical death-promoting Western diet to an "optimal" longevity diet can *add ten years--one entire decade--to their "healthy life expectancy!"* Moreover a 20-year-old American male who switches to an optimal diet adds 13 years to his expected lifespan.

Further, science shows that diet-driven life spans continue to expand in both men and women even into advanced ages. By switching to an optimal diet, a 60-year-old American female can expect to gain an extra eight years of life and a 60-year-old American male, nearly nine extra years. Even at age 80, adopting an optimal or longevity diet predictably gives an American woman an extra 2.6 years of life and an American man, 3.8 extra years.

It is never too early or too late to add minutes, hours, days, or years to your existence by eating longevity foods, using the information in this book as your guide. Nor do you need to make radical or exotic diet changes to increase your longevity. Researchers know that the most potent longevity foods are common legumes, whole grains, and nuts, and that the deadliest saboteurs of a long life are red and processed meats, refined grains, and sugar-sweetened beverages.

The potential longevity you gain from even slightly modifying your food choices is a scientific dream come true! Slowing down your aging process by choosing specific foods is not a dream, but a powerful reality.

Why This Book is Unlike Others

This groundbreaking book uniquely answers the vital question:" If I want to live as long as possible in reasonably good health, which foods does science say I should eat and avoid? This is the first book known to the author, to specifically present the latest scientific research identifying which food choices can help you reach your ultimate possible age.

Clearly if you eat foods shown to encourage longevity and discourage death, you are likely to age more slowly and live longer. Thus, this book gives you the latest dietary knowledge enabling you to live the longest healthiest life possible.

Most important: this book is based on impeccable science. The author is a lifelong medical journalist who uses only the highest quality scientific sources from world-class academic and professional researchers. Key research articles cited in this book can be verified and accessed through the National Library of Medicine's website and are presented in an Appendix Bibliography of this book.

How Specific Foods, Drinks, Diets, & Other Food Factors Affect Longevity

APPLE

Adds One-Third to Life Expectancy

If you believe the old adage "An apple a day keeps the doctor away," just listen to this latest claim: "Women over age 70 who eat an apple a day can expect *to live one third longer*!" It comes from Dr Jonathan Hodgson at the University of Western Australia. He actually did a study tracking 1400 women for 15 years and discovered that women who ate an apple a day did live *a remarkable 35 percent longer than those who did not eat apples.*

Indeed, science confirms that apples more than live up to their awesome reputation for stretching longevity. Other international research concluded that eating a mere *half an apple* a day slashed death risk as much as 20 percent in men and 43 percent in women of various ages.

A large Italian study documented that an apple a day dramatically slashes the odds of cancer. Specifically, a daily apple cuts the risk of prostate cancer by seven percent, of the esophagus by 22 percent, breast and ovarian by 24 percent, colon by 30 percent and the larynx by 41 percent. Smokers and former smokers who ate the most apples compared to the least had a lower risk of lung cancer.

A ten-year Swedish study found a decidedly reduced risk of stroke among 75,000 men and women who ate the most apples, versus the least.

Active Agents Researchers credit apple's high concentrations of flavonoid antioxidants, 50 percent of which are in the *apple's skin or peel.*

Essential Advice: *Eat an apple a day, being sure to include the peel. Wash apples well to remove waxy coating that may contain pesticides.*

AVOCADO

Boosts Heart Functioning

After three decades of studying avocadoes, Harvard researchers decreed these high-fat marvels (80 percent of calories in fat) to be a unique longevity force. Among 100,000 older Americans, those who ate avocados twice a week had a 15 to 22 percent *lower risk* of cardiovascular death than those who ignored avocadoes.

Avocado eaters also have higher good-type high density lipoprotein (HDL), as well as smaller waists, lower body mass index (BMI) and lower weight than non-avocado eaters.

Moreover, avocadoes are fierce antagonists of cancer. A recent study found that eating avocados only once a week depressed overall risk of cancer in men by 15 percent, and specifically bladder cancer by 28 percent and colorectal and lung cancer by 29 percent. Eating avocado also discourages the spread of prostate cancer cells.

The biggest avocado surprise comes from University of Kansas scientists who discovered that avocados actually *boost memory in old age.* People over age 60 who regularly eat avocados scored significantly higher on tests of cognition, particularly on *memory performance* tests, than non-avocado eaters. This is hugely important since memory decline is the most common complaint due to aging.

Active Agents: The magic ingredients in avocadoes are lutein, a strong antioxidant, and a high concentration of monounsaturated fats known to have anti-inflammatory and anti-cancer activity.

Essential Advice: *Eat half an avocado a day or at least three avocados a week.*

BANANA

Discourages Cancer

Called "exotic" until around 1900, bananas are now the most popular fruit in the world, including the United States. Americans eat about 27 pounds a year. Most banana lovers eat them ripe, but, surprisingly, much of a banana's longevity factor is also found in unripe green bananas.

In 2022 international scientists were surprised to discover incredibly strong anti-cancer activity in a unique type of fiber, called "resistant starch." mainly on full display in unripe green bananas. During digestion the fiber is not broken down and is left to ferment in the large intestine. As the banana fully ripens, the resistant starch diminishes or disappears.

Volunteers who ate a daily dose of resistant starch comparable to that in a slightly green banana every day for two years reduced their risk of various cancers by 50-60 percent! Over a decade only five new cases of upper gastrointestinal (GI) cancers occurred in 463 participants who consumed the resistant starch compared with 21 cancer cases in the 455 who took a placebo. Resistant starch was most apt to deter esophageal, gastric, pancreatic, and duodenal cancers, but not colorectal cancers. The anti-cancer protection lasted ten years after patients stopped taking banana-like resistant starch.

Resistant starch also improves insulin sensitivity by up to 50 percent, cutting the risk of type 2 diabetes, obesity, heart disease and dementia.

Active Agents: Unripe green bananas provide 21 grams of resistant starch in 3.5 ounces-- compared with only one gram in ripe bananas. Ripe bananas are bursting with more antioxidants.

Essential Advice: *Eat three or four bananas or plantains a week, both raw and ripe, as well as slightly green and cooked. Put green bananas and cooked green plantains in smoothies.*

BEANS & LEGUMES

Universal Champions

Beans are utterly unglamorous. Yet science unequivocally anoints the lowly bean as "the world's ultimate longevity food." Virtually every longevity diet in the world prominently features dried beans or the broader family called legumes as a must. Technically, legumes include beans, lentils, peas, and peanuts.

Undeniably, beans are the one food eaten by inhabitants of the world's so-designated "Blue Zones" where centenarians tend to congregate. Eating one half to three fourths of a cup of cooked beans a day can depress your risk of dying by 16 percent, according to international consensus. Yet less than five percent of Americans eat legumes every day. Sadly, only one third eat legumes as often as once a month!

Our legume deficiency has deadly consequences. According to Dan Buettner, founder of the longevity organization named Blue Zones: "Legumes are the cornerstone of a typical centenarian's diet. They are a longevity all-star food. If you're eating about a cup of beans a day, it's probably worth an extra four years of life expectancy."

One recent study showed that the mortality risk dropped seven to eight percent for every one-third of a cup of beans seniors ate. People who said they never ate beans undeniably had far higher death rates than bean eaters.

Active agents: Dried beans, lentils, black-eyed peas, split peas are packed with both insoluble and soluble fiber, credited with much of their longevity activity.

Essential Advice: *If you do nothing else to extend your life, eat beans, lentils or peas and peanuts (all in the legume family) every day or at least a few times a week.*

BEER

Dilutes Life Expectancy

Beer, the most widely consumed alcoholic beverage in the world, has existed for thousands of years and may seem less noxious because its alcohol is diluted. But, in excess beer is the same threat to longevity as other alcoholic beverages. Beer drinking is decidedly linked to "a higher risk of early death, alcohol dependence or alcohol use disorder, depression, liver disease, weight gain and cancers," according to substantial evidence.

Male bingers in Finland who typically drank six or more bottles of beer in one session had triple the risk of premature death and six times the odds of fatal heart attack as men who drank half that or three bottles at one time. A study in Louisiana linked higher beer consumption to 24 percent of all premature deaths in the state's larger cities.

Strong evidence shows that drinking more than one daily beer *increases* your chances of both ischemic and hemorrhagic strokes.

Beer, like other alcoholic beverages, also stimulates cancer. The more alcohol you drink, the greater your odds of developing cancers of the oral cavity, colon, liver, and breast. Even moderate drinking is associated with 30,000 to 40,000 cancer deaths a year.

Definitely do not follow the advice of one highly publicized Italian study suggesting that "moderate" beer drinking—up to one beer daily for women and two for men--actually reduces cardiovascular disease.

Active Agents: Alcohol is the main villain in beer.

Essential Advice: *Best advice is to restrict beer to no more than one pint a day, and preferably less or none. Research suggests that every excess pint beyond a daily pint shaves half an hour off the life expectancy of men age 40.*

BEET

Revs Up Brain Energy

The ancient Greeks and Romans viewed beets as a universal cure-all. Modern medicine agrees that the bulb and juice exhibit profound effects on blood flow. University of London research found that a daily cup of beetroot juice can reduce systolic and diastolic blood pressure as much as pharmaceutical drugs and may cut the risk of fatal heart disease and stroke by seven and ten percent respectively.

Beets' magical chemistry is widely known. Beets possess the highest concentration of sodium nitrates of any edible plant. (Other high-nitrate plants are leafy greens, spinach and celery.) In the digestive tract, nitrates convert to nitric oxide, a kind of high-powered performance drug.

Male cyclists who drank 17 ounces of high-nitrate beetroot juice improved performance by three percent. Female kayakers who downed two shots of beet juice (about 300 mg of nitrate) improved performance by two percent. Runners ran faster after eating whole beets.

Especially fascinating is the power of beets, along with other nitrate-packed foods, to rev up blood flow in aging brains. Scientists at Wake Forest University measured the blood flow in specific brain regions of subjects over age 75 after they ate both high-and low-nitrate diets. Brain scans clearly revealed *improved* blood flow in frontal lobe white matter involved in executive functioning in older adults after they consumed high-nitrate foods, such as beets.

Active Agents: Sodium nitrate in beet bulbs.

Essential Advice: *Eat a cup of beets or beet juice daily or a few hours preceding physical or mental activity to slightly improve blood flow, performance and prolong life.*

BERRIES

Amazing Defenders Against Death

Of 400 different types of berries, many have impressive longevity powers. Most common among the powerful are acai berries, blueberries, raspberries, blackberries, cranberries and strawberries, with blueberries ranked number one. In an analysis of nearly two million women, those who ate blueberries more than once a week reduced their risk of dying by 33 percent! Strawberries were a close second.

When tested separately from the whole berry, specific blueberry chemical constituents lowered odds of fatal strokes by 37 percent and fatal cardiovascular disease by 18 percent.

Among a group of middle-aged Norwegian men, those who ate the most berries of any kind compared to the least had 12 percent lower chances of dying from any cause.

Parkinson's disease patients who ate berries and other flavonoid-rich foods three times a week had 70 percent lower death rates than those eating such foods once a week or less.

A recent medical review of common berries revealed these facts: Blueberries have twice the life-extending flavonoids as raspberries and strawberries. Cranberries have strong antioxidant activity contributing to longevity. Blueberries, strawberries, and raspberries demonstrate anti-cancer activity. Strawberries fight obesity and cardiovascular risk and may also lower Alzheimer's risk in the elderly.

Active Agents: All berries are packed to varying degrees with anthocyanins, or flavonoids, a pigment in the outer skin of berries, credited as the main source of their longevity-promoting activity.

Essential Advice: *Eat fresh raw, heated, frozen, and thawed berries; all have super-high antioxidant capacity and formidable death-defying activity.*

BEVERAGES with ALCOHOL

Unsafe Sip by Sip

Until recently science agreed that a little alcohol won't kill you and might be beneficial. Updated advice now says that even a little alcohol can sabotage longevity.

Most alarming, even a sip more than one alcoholic drink a day may shorten life, concluded a 2018 worldwide study of 600,000 current drinkers in the medical journal *Lancet.* That means no more than a 12-ounce beer, 8-ounce glass of wine or ounce of spirits in a 24-hour period.

The sobering news from many studies is that the more alcohol ingested, the more your life expectancy shrinks. From two to three and a half drinks a day brings death two years prematurely. Four or more daily drinks attracts death four to five years earlier.

Indeed, every additional alcoholic drink a day cuts your life short by at least 30 minutes, according to convincing research.

In fact, research has revealed 38 percent higher death rates in former drinkers than in life-time teetotalers. Worst of all is binge drinking. Four to five drinks within two hours more than *doubles* your odds of early death over a period of two decades.

True, a few outlier studies suggest that abstainers occasionally have higher death rates than moderate drinkers. However, here's the truest universal bottom line from world-prominent researchers writing in the prestigious medical journal Lancet: *"Our results show that the safest level of drinking is none."*

Active Agents: Ethanol, the intoxicating addictive agent in beer, wine and distilled spirits is a major cause of death.

Essential Advice: *For greatest life expectancy, avoid alcohol. Or at least limit alcohol to seven ounces of wine, one beer or one fluid ounce of spirits daily.*

BLUE ZONES DIET

Ideal for Centenarians

There are five so-called *Blue Zones* in the world where people consistently reach age 100 in good health. In his best-selling book, *The Blue Zones Solution*, author Dan Buettner lists the world's five longevity hot spots and their typical diets.

1. **Ikaria, Greece** has "*One of the world's lowest rates of middle-age mortality.*" Diet: olive oil, greens, arugula, potatoes (not fried), feta cheese, chickpeas, whole lemons, coffee, honey, herbal tea.

2. **Okinawa, Japan** is "*Home to the world's longest-lived women.*" Diet: Bitter melons, tofu, sweet potatoes, garlic, turmeric, brown rice, green tea, shiitake mushrooms, seaweed.

3. **Sardinia** is "*Home to the world's highest concentration of centenarian men.*" Diet: Goat's milk, sourdough and high-fiber bread, barley, fennel bulb, almonds, chickpeas, tomatoes, red wine.

4. **Loma Linda, California** has "*A high population of Seventh Day Adventists, who exceed the*

average American lifespan by ten years." Diet: Avocados, salmon, nuts, soy, beans, oatmeal, whole wheat bread.

5. **Costa *Rica (Nicoya Peninsula*)** has the "W*orld's lowest rates of middle age mortality and many centenarian*s." Diet: Corn tortillas, squash, papayas, yams, black beans, bananas, palm tree fruit.

The so-called *Blue Zones Diet* consists of mainly plants, minimal meat regarded as "a side dish," three ounces of fish three times a week, goat milk, nut snacks, no dairy, beans every day, natural sugars in fruits, whole grain and sourdough bread, coffee, tea and wine in moderation, no chips, pastries, cookies.

.

Essential Advice: *For a longevity blueprint, mimic these five diets that are prominent among populations living in centenarian blue zones.*

BREAD

White is Death's Best Friend

The path to an early grave is paved with white bread. The more white bread you eat, the more likely your demise, according to a 2021 landmark study of 137, 000 people in 21 countries by Canadian professors at McMaster University and published in the prestigious *British Medical Journal.*

The study revealed for the first time the enormous lethal and largely unacknowledged hazards of white bread. Eating seven slices of white bread a day, compared to two slices, multiplied death risk by 27 percent. Eating white bread also increased death odds 33 percent for cardiovascular disease, 31 percent for non-cardiovascular disease and 47 percent for strokes! White bread's fatal flaw: It's made from "refined" grains, stripped of all-important fiber and nutrients.

Further, numerous studies identify white bread as a prime cancer threat. Its basic ingredient, "refined white flour" *increases* the risk of colon and gastric cancer. In contrast, "unrefined" whole grains baked into bread *reduce* the comparative risk of colorectal, colon gastric, pancreatic, and esophageal cancer. *In one impressive long-term study, cancer probabilities fell six to 12 percent after eating half a slice to three slices per day of whole grain bread rather than white bread.*

Another monumental sin of white bread: when digested, it behaves like sugar by spiking blood glucose and raising the risk of type 2 diabetes. as well as other sugar-related diseases.

Essential Advice: *Avoid white bread when possible. Eat breads made from wheat, rye, barley, corn, etc. Look for "100% whole grain" labels. Also ok for seekers of longevity: sourdough bread which is fermented.*

BREAKFAST

Skipping Brings Death Sooner

Science is firmly in favor of eating breakfast. Texas Tech University researchers followed over 7,000 middle aged Americans for 22 years. Sixteen percent rarely ate breakfast; 23 percent ate breakfast on some days, and 61 percent ate breakfast every day. The bottom line was startling: *Those who rarely ate breakfast were 50 per cent more apt to die of cancer and 69 percent more apt to die sooner than those who ate breakfast every day.*

Equally disturbing, new research at the University of Iowa ties skipping breakfast to fatal cardiovascular disease. *Individuals who did not eat breakfast were forty percent more likely to die of heart disease than those who ate breakfast! The breakfast skippers were also 12 percent more apt to die earlier.*

University of Michigan researchers reported that adult males who did not eat breakfast had less vigor and higher depression scores. Women breakfast-skippers felt more anxious and fatigued. Extensive research links not eating breakfast to a multitude of other problems, including obesity, troubled sleep, vitamin D deficiency, higher consumption of empty calories, high blood pressure, and chronic stress.

Other research shows that those who ate breakfast less than once a week were twice as likely to attempt suicide as daily breakfast eaters. In another study, college students who ate breakfast every day, had the "highest happiness score."

Essential Advice: *Be sure to eat something for breakfast every morning. Suggestions: whole grain cereals, including oats, as well as nuts, blueberries or other fruit, coffee, and tea. Eggs occasionally may not kill you but skip the bacon and other meats.*

BUTTER & MARGARINE

Longevity Detractors

Butter may not be as deadly as you fear, nor margarine as lifesaving. Top food and nutrition experts have argued over butter vs margarine for several decades. There was a sigh of relief among nutrition opinion-makers after a 2016 Tufts University study of 636,000 participants pronounced butter "neutral"—not likely to make any difference either way in your risk of death, or of cardiovascular disease or diabetes.

But the alarm blared again in 2021, reviving concern, after a NIH-AARP study of half a million elderly Americans revealed that those who ate the most butter, compared to the least, had *nine per cent higher* death rates over a 16-year period. Eating the most butter also was linked to 18 percent higher death odds from diabetes. High margarine eaters fared only slightly better, with 12 percent higher overall death rates.

Butter also spiked higher death rates from cardiovascular disease, cancer, respiratory disease, kidney disease and chronic liver disease. Margarine was linked to higher death risk from respiratory disease and kidney disease.

The alarming bottom line: A daily tablespoon of butter is reported to raise overall death rates by seven percent and a daily tablespoon of margarine, by four percent.

Recent Harvard research presents the ideal solution: substitute olive oil for butter and margarine. When researchers substituted olive oil for equal amounts of butter or margarine in a huge health professional's study of 28 years, deaths from all causes dropped an astonishing twenty percent!

Active Agents: Villains are presumably high saturated fat in butter and artificial chemicals in margarine.

Essential Advice: *Skip both butter and margarine and /or substitute olive oil when appropriate.*

CABBAGE

Spectacular Life Preserver

In ancient Rome, cabbage was used as a panacea to cure virtually all diseases. Today leading scientists point to cabbage--red, purple, white, and green--as a potential antidote to deadly covid 19, as well as other chronic maladies including cancer. Dr Jean Bousquet at Montpelier University declares that *"Eating sauerkraut, coleslaw and raw cabbage could protect against the coronavirus."*

He says eating plain cabbage cuts covid death odds 11 percent, and that sauerkraut or Kimchi slashes covid fatality risk 35 percent, and helps prevent chronic inflammation, the world's leading cause of death. Cabbage is also a cruciferous vegetable with additional virtues. One European study claimed that increasing cabbage consumption by a mere one gram per day (1/28th of a single ounce) could reduce a country's mortality rate by 13 percent.

The National Institutes of Health discovered cabbage's peculiar anti-cancer powers in the 1980's, revealing that eating cabbage once or more a week cuts the chances of deadly pancreatic cancer by 38 percent!

Other Chicago-based research confirmed one-third lower breast cancer odds in women who eat raw or lightly cooked cabbage and sauerkraut more than four times a week versus less than twice a week. In another study, eating cabbage helped prevent and treat type 2 diabetes.

Active Agents: All cabbage varieties possess antioxidant activity, but red cabbage surpasses not only all cabbages, but a dozen other cruciferous vegetables!

Essential Advice: *Eat cabbage raw or lightly cooked and also as sauerkraut and kimchi a couple of times a week. For greatest potency, choose red cabbage, followed by Chinese white and green cabbage.*

CAFFEINE

Keeps You Awake and Alive!

Sixty four percent of American adults get a daily longevity kick from caffeine. And 70 percent of it comes from coffee. The rest comes from tea, sodas, energy drinks, and chocolate, for a daily average of 165 milligrams of caffeine.

When American scientists compared caffeine intake with death rates in 23,878 individuals over age 20, they discovered that a daily intake of 200 milligrams of caffeine, (about two cups of coffee) cut death risk significantly, notably from cardiovascular disease.

In a striking University of California study, Americans who consumed 100 to 399 milligrams of caffeine a day (one to four cups of caffeinated coffee) were *ten percent less likely to die of anything* than those who consumed a mere 50 milligrams.

In a large 2022 study, overweight caffeine consumers who consumed *moderate* amounts of caffeine had 25 percent lower death odds. In those with *high* caffeine intake, death rates dropped 47 percent.

However, people vary widely in their individual tolerance to caffeine. It can increase anxiety, raise blood pressure, cause heart and sleeping problems, as well as withdrawal headaches, fatigue and depression, and should be restricted by sensitive individuals.

Active Agents: Caffeine has strong antioxidant activity which is thought to be its most important pro-longevity feature.

Essential Advice: The Food and Drug Administration declares 400 milligrams of daily caffeine "safe" for adults, or about four cups of brewed coffee. Harvard experts say pregnant women should limit caffeine to under 200 milligrams daily, and children under age twelve should avoid high caffeine foods and beverages altogether.

Common Sources of Caffeine: Eight ounces of brewed coffee, 100 mg caffeine; instant coffee, 60 mg; decaf, 4 mg; espresso 1.5 ounce shot, 65 mg; black tea, 47 mg; green tea, 28 mg; decaf tea, 2 mg; herbal tea, zero; 12-ounce soda, regular or diet, 40 mg; Mountain Dew, 55 mg; 1 ounce dark chocolate, 24 mg; milk chocolate, 6 mg; 16-ounce energy drinks, 170 mg.

CALORIES

Overloads Destroy Longevity

It's well known that reducing calories in lab animals by 30 to 50 percent without causing malnutrition, suppresses chronic diseases and increases animals' lifespan by thirty to fifty percent! So, shouldn't the same thing happen in humans, making calorie cutting a pathway to longevity?

Yes, says Dr. Luigi Fontana, adjunct professor of medicine at Washington University, and pioneer researcher on calorie restriction and longevity. His research shows that restricting calories can reduce inflammation (a promoter of aging and age-related chronic diseases), slow aging of the heart, prevent insulin resistance and improve heart functioning.

Practitioners of caloric restriction, compared to high calorie-consumers, often are reported to have the heart functioning of someone 20 years younger, and a 50 percent lower risk of coronary heart disease.

Restricting calories also reduces blood markers in humans for risk of prostate, breast and colon cancer.

Increased longevity due to calorie deprivation was particularly evident in statistics from World War II. As food shortages worsened in wartime Denmark, death rates plunged 34 percent. Similarly, food cutbacks in Norway translated into a 30 per cent dive in mortality rates. Japanese inhabitants of Okinawa after the war who ate 46 percent fewer calories than US residents saw cardiac death rates drop by an astonishing 87 percent.

Experts say without doubt that caloric restriction can reduce risk of cancer, diabetes, heart disease, obesity, type 2 diabetes and delay biological aging and death in humans.

Essential Advice: *Although theoretically cutting calories may keep you alive longer, it is obviously tricky. Don't severely cut calories without consulting a dietician, doctor or other professional to be sure you do not accidentally do yourself more harm than good.*

CANDY

Death's Faithful Accomplice

Americans eat more candy than any other nation, 25 pounds per person per year, surpassing China, Germany, Russia, and the United Kingdom.

Harvard investigators sought to find out how candy consumption affects longevity in a memorable study of 7841 middle-aged male alumni in 1998. The results were unexpected, shocking, and literally unbelievable. Men who ate candy a few times a week lived nearly a year *longer* than men who shunned candy. At a loss to explain the bizarre anointment of candy as longevity food, researchers credited atypically high amounts of antioxidant rich chocolate in the men's candy allotment.

The mistake was soon contradicted and corrected by a subsequent 15-year Harvard study, indicting candy as quite hazardous to health.

The obvious fatal flaw in all candy is its inevitable massive amounts of "added sugar" that promotes inflammation and destruction of the heart. As revealed by the more recent Harvard investigation, individuals who ate 17 to 21 percent of their calories as "added sugar" compared to eight percent, *were 38 percent more apt to die of cardiovascular disease.*

Researchers further warn that the higher your intake of "added sugar" the more likely you are to die of heart disease, as well as to suffer strokes, type 2 diabetes, obesity and damage to your pancreas and kidneys. *Added sugar, the major ingredient of candy, is a formidable premiere killer worldwide.*

Active Agents*:* Added sugar accounts for 70 percent of calories in some candy. The more added sugar, the deadlier the candy.

Essential Advice*: Eat candy sparingly. Probably the worst: candy corn which is pure sugar. The least harmful: dark chocolate, lower in sugar and higher in certain life-stretching phytochemicals. For maximum longevity, it makes sense to curtail candy consumption.*

CARBOHYDRATES

They Mess with Mortality

Carbohydrates can either prolong your life or kill you early depending on their source and quantity. Research reveals that both splurging on and restricting high-carb foods can cut life short.

Normally Americans get 45 to 65 percent of their daily calories from carbohydrates. Eating more or less than that is a prescription for premature death.

In a recent definitive study of 432,179 participants, Harvard researchers found that death rates shot up about 20 percent in people who ate both less than 40 percent of their calories and more than 70 percent of their calories in carbs. *Those most likely to live the longest ate from 50 to 55 percent—or about half their calories in carbohydrates.*

However, also critical is which foods you choose to replace carbohydrates when you restrict them. For example, if you go on a low- carbohydrate diet and replace the carbs with *animal-derived* protein, such as meat, your likelihood of death rises, whereas if you replace the carbs with plant-derived protein or fat, for example, legumes, your odds of death decrease and you're apt to survive longer.

Further, eating so-called simple or refined carbs, mainly sugar, unlike complex carbs, spikes death rates.

Death-promoting simple carbs include white bread, pasta, cookies, cake, candy, and sugar-sweetened beverages. Complex *death-defying carbs* include whole grains, fruits, vegetables, milk, nuts, seeds, legumes (beans, lentils, peas).

Essential Advice: *To live longest in good health, eat about half of your calories in complex carbohydrates. Avoid or restrict simple refined carbohydrates, known as sugar.*

CARROT

Formidable Foe of Cancer

The evidence is in your blood. After you eat carrots, your blood levels of alpha and beta carotene, an orange pigment, as well as vitamin C and other phytochemicals, rise. And your chances of death from any cause, including cancer, drop at least 20 percent. Both carotene and vitamin C exhibit strong anti-cancer activity.

Carrots and carotenes have a long history of deterring cancer. A 1986 Swedish study first identified carrots as a dietary barrier to pancreatic cancer, a lethal smoking-related cancer. Individuals with the lowest beta carotene blood levels versus the highest were also four times more apt to develop lung cancer.

A string of recent studies cements carrots' strong anti-cancer reputation. A 2020 international study showed that those who ate the most carrots compared with the least had an astonishing 40 percent lower risk of lung cancer. Another new study linked high consumption of carrots to a 26 percent reduction in gastric or stomach cancer.

An analysis of more than 100,000 Chinese in 2022 found that eating moderate amounts of carrots reduced incidence and deaths from colorectal cancer by 21 percent. Carrots thwart the spread of urothelial cancer, related to the urethra and bladder. High blood levels of beta carotene, a strong antioxidant in carrots, predicted a five percent drop in risk of breast cancer.

Active Agents: Carrots are rich in carotenes and vitamin A and C, all shown to have strong antioxidant anti-cancer activity.

Essential Advice: *Make it a habit of eating carrots raw and lightly cooked. A cup a day, or more infuses your bloodstream with longevity promoting chemicals.*

CELERY

Mimic the Man with a Juicer

Occasionally medical journals present evidence based on an individual case, rather than on a larger group study. Such is a case report published in the June 2021 issue of *Journal of Chiropractic Medicine* about a 74-year-old man with hypertension who treated it by drinking celery juice.

Previously he had tried three different blood pressure drugs which did not control his blood pressure and produced serious side effects, sending him to a hospital emergency room twice. He quit taking the drugs and agreed to only one lifestyle change suggested by someone on his medical team: to start drinking celery juice.

Using a common-brand juicer, he liquified ten to twelve stalks of celery which he drank every morning in addition to his regular diet. In the first month his systolic blood pressure dropped about 10 mm Hg. In the next six months on daily celery juice his systolic blood pressure sank about 32 mm Hg to a low of 120 mm. His diastolic blood pressure fell a couple of points. His blood pressure readings, now reduced to normal, were taken by medical personnel.

The authors of the study say it is impossible to know whether the celery juice alone so dramatically reduced his blood pressure, but they note that celery seed extracts and phytochemicals have slashed blood pressure in both animal and human subjects in lab tests.

Active Agents: Celery contains a slew of super antioxidants, including caffeic acid, ferulic acid, tannin, saponin and kaempferol.

Essential Advice: *It makes sense to eat celery and celery juice regularly since there is convincing evidence it dampens blood pressure and prolongs life.*

CEREAL

Choose Lifesavers Not Killers

With the dawn of the twentieth century came new-fangled foods called corn flakes, grape-nuts, and shredded wheat, etc. Today Americans gobble up twenty billion dollars' worth of ready-to-eat cold cereals a year. As a longevity food, they are a mixed blessing.

The power of cereals to discourage numerous chronic diseases, and prevent death are substantial, as revealed in a recent National Institutes of Health study of 367,442 Americans. The study showed that eating the most ready- to- eat cereals compared to the least slashed overall death rates by *15 percent.* Further, the most enthusiastic cereal eaters were ten to 30 percent less apt to die of cardiovascular disease, cancer, diabetes, and other chronic diseases.

Another huge study in twenty-one countries, published in the *British Medical Journal* in 2021 by University of Toronto researchers echoed the good, but stressed that the type of cereal—refined or whole grain—is critical. In this massive study, eating the most "refined" cereals meaning the whole grain is demolished, compared to the least refined, *actually raised death rates by 27 percent*! Such refined cereals typically have high sugar and low fiber and should be avoided.

So, eating just any cereal is not advisable. Eat only ready-to-eat cereals with at least five grams of fiber and fewer than 2.5 grams of added sugar per serving. Examples: Fiber One has the highest fiber of 18 grams per serving and original Shredded Wheat has 8 grams of fiber; both have no sugar.

Active Agents: Researchers attribute most of cereal's longevity activity to its high fiber.

Essential Advice. *Read labels and eat only whole grain cereals with high fiber, no or low added sugar, and low sodium. Avoid refined ready - to - eat -cereals. Also eat hot whole grain cereals, including oatmeal.*

CHEESE

Not Likely the Kiss of Death

Fermenting milk to make cheese began thousands of years ago. But whether cheese, especially high fat, is more apt to expand life, promote premature death or is life-and-death neutral is far from scientifically settled. Studies give widely varying answers of yes, no and maybe. In short, science is all over the place about how good or bad cheese is for your longevity.

A 2019 study of a thousand elderly Dutch showed that eating three quarters of an ounce of cheese a day had *no impact* on mortality; it did not deter or hasten death.

The famed Karolinska Institution tracked 80,000 Swedish middle-aged men and women for 18 years and found *no connection* between eating any amount of cheese and risk of stroke, fatal or nonfatal.

Scientists at the University of Reading in the United Kingdom who analyzed 29 worldwide studies with a million participants in a massive investigation of cheese and health, concluded that people *who eat more* *cheese do <u>not</u> increase their risk of heart disease, strokes, or death from any cause.*

In a few studies, eating cheese seemed to raise death rates by one to two percent. One outlier study did link cheese with a 23 per cent higher risk of fatal cancer.

And, yes, an equally rare finding emerged from research at the University of Reading: It suggested that eating a large bite of cheese daily (one-third of an ounce) actually *reduced* the risk of death by two percent.

Active Agents: Fermentation changes milk into cheese.

Essential Advice: *Since the death risk from cheese is somewhat contradictory but seems mostly neutral, it seems inappropriate to splurge on it or avoid it entirely. Somewhat cautious and moderate seems a safer way to go until science comes up with more consistent advice.*

CHILI PEPPERS

Red Hot Life Extenders

Scientists at the University of Vermont College of Medicine recently reported that among 16,000 Americans, those who ate the most hot chili peppers were 13 percent less apt to die prematurely than those who never ate hot peppers.

This is not peculiar to Americans. It's a worldwide phenomenon. Harvard and Chinese nutritionists recently tracked the diets of half a million Chinese, focusing on their consumption of fresh and dried chili peppers, chili sauce and chili oil. Undeniable conclusion: Those who ate hot peppers almost every day, compared with less than once a week, were 14 percent less likely to die of any cause.

At least half a dozen other studies worldwide link hot spicy foods to a lower risk of various cancers, obesity, cardiovascular disease, diabetes. and death. Experts credit hot spicy food's benefits mostly to its main ingredient, capsaicin, (responsible for the spicy sensation) that can affect the regulation of systolic and diastolic blood pressure and insulin resistance.

Some people avoid chili peppers, fearing they instigate or aggravate heartburn, but experts say the evidence is far from conclusive. Nor is there convincing evidence that chili peppers cause stomach cancer although one study suggested a connection.

Active Agents: Capsaicin, the main source of "hot" in chili peppers, has strong anti-obesity, antioxidant, anti-inflammatory, and anti-hypertensive activity.

Essential Advice: *Eat hot chili peppers twice a week or more, including fresh jalapeno, serrano, bird's eye, and habanero peppers. It may help stop the mouth "burn" of hot peppers to drink a glass of whole milk but don't overdo it.*

CHOCOLATE

Super-Food with a Dark Side

Chocolate has spectacular longevity powers, as revealed by a 30-year American-European study of 27,000 men in 2021, tracking how much chocolate they ate and how long they lived. Men who averaged a mere half an ounce a day of chocolate lived 9 to 12 percent longer than men who ate no chocolate. Further, those eating the most compared to the least chocolate, were 20 percent less apt to die from coronary heart disease, and 13 percent less likely to die from cancer.

So powerful is chocolate that death rates fell steadily in the above study until chocolate consumption dropped below two grams daily, half a chocolate tidbit. Recent Harvard research also reported that a couple of cups of chocolate's antioxidant flavanols cut cardiovascular disease risk by a stunning 27 percent among 20,000 older Americans.

Unfortunately, *dark* chocolate, the only type worth eating, is often contaminated with potentially toxic cadmium and/or lead. In a recent test, 100 percent of

23 dark chocolates had high cadmium and lead, compared with only three or 13 percent of milk chocolates, causing experts to warn that a single daily ounce of dark chocolate could be unsafe. Fortunately, the longevity benefits of dark chocolate kick in after eating a m*ere one third of an ounce a day,*

Active Agents: Dark chocolate's main longevity boost is due to its high content of antioxidants called flavanols, which are far lower in milk chocolate and zero in white chocolate.

Essential Advice: *Experts say it's ok to eat one or two ounces of dark chocolate throughout the day or two-thirds of an ounce of milk chocolate. As for white chocolate, don't bother. It has high sugar and zero real chocolate. Of course, chocolate's risk is heightened when sugar is added to make candy.*

COFFEE

Sure Bet to Boost Longevity

Drinking two to five cups of coffee a day may cut your risk of type 2 diabetes, heart disease, liver and endometrial cancers, Parkinson's disease, depression, and delay death, according to Frank Hu, chair of Harvard Medical School's department of Nutrition.

Specifically, half a cup of coffee a day cut death odds five percent; a full daily cup decreased odds nine percent and two daily cups slashed death risk by a remarkable 18 percent. Drinking more, up to 7.5 cups a day did not further increase longevity.

Coffee especially seems to delay premature cardiovascular deaths. Two and a half cups a day slashed fatal heart disease odds by 17 percent and deadly diabetes risk by 29 percent. Six and a half daily cups cut death odds from respiratory disease by 28 percent.

One study reported that two daily cups of coffee reduced odds of fatal cancer by four percent, and remarkably, so did drinking four times that much or seven and a half cups daily. This suggests that the optimal anti-cancer dose for coffee is a mere couple of cups a day.

Research also finds that after six daily regular coffees, longevity ceases to rise further, and ill effects may begin to kick in. Excessive caffeinated coffee can cause or aggravate anxiety, insomnia, heartburn, and increased heart rate.

Which type coffee is most apt to increase life span? In a 12-year international study of nearly half a million people, two to three daily cups of instant coffee reduced death odds by 11 percent compared with 14 percent for decaf coffee and 27 percent for regular ground coffee.

Active Agents*: Important: R*esearchers attribute most of coffee's life-enhancing powers to non-caffeine constituents, so don't dismiss decaf, nor suffer needlessly trying to overcome caffeine intolerance.

Essential Advice: *Two to five daily cups of coffee appear safe and/or beneficial for most adults. Go easy with added cream or sugar. Restrict coffee if it causes distress, insomnia, upset stomach or if you are pregnant or breast-feeding.*

The American Academy of Pediatrics recommends no caffeinated coffee for children under twelve and less than one cup a day for adolescents between twelve and eighteen.

Also experts suggest brewing coffee with a paper filter because unfiltered coffee is associated with higher rates of early death.

CORN

Old World Pro-Life Staple

Christopher Columbus discovered corn in America in 1492 and spread the word, helping make corn one of our most popular longevity foods.

Corn is actually not a vegetable; it's a whole grain with unique powers to ward off cardiovascular disease, type 2 diabetes, obesity, digestive diseases and cancer, mainly of the breast, esophagus, stomach and prostate. In lab tests, for example, purple corn and tortillas discourage the spread of prostate and breast cancer.

Further, subjects who ate two and a half daily servings of whole grains, including corn meal and popcorn, were 21 percent less apt to develop cardiovascular disease than those eating only half a daily serving. A huge Harvard study of 118,085 health professionals revealed that each extra serving of whole grain corn and popcorn further decreased rates of cardiovascular disease.

Swapping other high carb foods for high fiber corn decreases fat accumulation and obesity. The phytochemicals in corn also reduce the risk of insulin resistance and type 2 diabetes. High-fiber corn bran muffins dramatically increased feelings of satiety and discouraged weight gain. By the way, corn does not aggravate diverticular disease, say researchers.

Active Agents: Experts credit corn's super high antioxidant activity—exceeding that of rice, wheat and oats—for its longevity activity, along with resistant starch, a form of insoluble fiber.

Essential Advice: *Eat corn of all colors--yellow, red, blue, purple, and black. Each provides varying types of beneficial phytochemicals, including antioxidants.*

CRUCIFEROUS VEGETABLES

Totems for a Long Life

Cruciferous vegetables, also called brassica, are a plant family with unique longevity powers. Its famous members include arugula, bok choy, broccoli, Brussels sprouts, cabbage, cauliflower, collard greens, kale, turnips, radishes, rutabaga, and watercress.

Although potency varies, all cruciferous vegetables have impeccable credentials for fending off death. A recent Japanese study found that men who ate the most cruciferous vegetables compared to the least were 14 percent less apt to die for any reason. In women, the overall death risk for enthusiastic cruciferous consumers is 11 percent lower than for crucifer abstainers.

Cruciferous vegetables consistently ward off cancer. A study at Roswell Park Comprehensive Cancer Center found that people who ate three cups of *raw* cruciferous vegetables a week compared with one and a half cups had an astonishing 45 percent drop in likelihood of death from pancreatic cancer. Eating *cooked* cruciferous vegetables cut pancreatic death risk by 50 percent!

Cruciferous vegetables also thwart deaths from gastric, lung and endometrial cancers. In studies women with lung cancer who ate the most cruciferous vegetables compared to the least survived 30 percent longer. Men with prostate cancer who ate the most crucifers, particularly broccoli and cauliflower once a week compared to once a month, cut their death chances nearly in half.

Active Agents: Unique phytochemicals in cruciferous vegetables called glucosinolates and isothiocyanates are strong antioxidants and antibiotics that resist cancer and premature aging.

Essential Advice: *It's super smart for survival and longevity to eat a cup of cruciferous vegetables a day, cooked or raw.*

DASH DIET

Famous Blood Pressure Downer

The DASH (Dietary Approaches to Stop Hypertension) diet is one of the most famous in the world. Introduced in 1997, it is proven as effective as blood pressure medications and regarded as a formidable lifesaver in a world where high blood pressure kills about ten million people a year. In 2023, the DASH Diet was voted the number one best diet for eight years in a row by US News and World Reports Magazine.

The DASH Diet is anointed by masses of meticulous research. The latest: New York's Beth Israel Deaconess Medical Center reported that the Dash Diet cut the 10-year risk of atherosclerotic cardiovascular disease by 10 percent and was twice as effective in women and four times more effective in Blacks as similar diets. It works especially well when combined with sodium reduction.

Moreover, a recent meta-analysis by Canadian scientists revealed that the DASH diet produced a 20 percent reduction in the risk of cardiovascular disease, strokes and diabetes. It also decreased blood glucose levels by 29 percent in subjects with type 2 diabetes.

Typically, the DASH Diet includes a daily four to five servings of whole grains, five servings of vegetables, two or three fruits, two low-fat dairy foods, one three-ounce serving of fish, poultry, or meat, two or three servings of unsaturated fats and oils and seven to eight servings a week of beans, nuts, or seeds.

The DASH diet is also very similar to the Mediterranean Diet.

Active Ingredients: Foods in the DASH diet are rich in potassium, calcium and magnesium, and low in sodium, saturated fat and added sugars.

Essential Advice: *Follow the DASH diet to delay damage from hypertension. This can add as much as a decade to your life if you begin the diet in early adulthood, or during your twenties.*

DIET SODAS

They Kill You, Too, But Faster

The startling truth is that artificially sweetened soft drinks, so-called "diet" sodas, are *about three times more likely to kill you* than regular sugar-sweetened high-calorie soft drinks. That's the conclusion of a large European study of 451,743 individuals, published in 2019 in the *Journal of the American Medical Association Internal Medicine.*

Specifically, two or more sugar-sweetened soft drinks a day boosted death odds by eight percent. The same amount of artificially sweetened drinks escalated the death risk by 26 percent!

Deaths related to diet soft drinks are primarily due to cardiovascular disease, and the more you drink, the greater your risk of death.

In a large Harvard study, older women who guzzled the most "diet drinks," compared to none or under one a week, had a 30 percent higher likelihood of stroke, and a 16 percent greater chance of dying. In heavier women with a body mass index over 30, the death risk from diet drinks doubled.

Cancer was also a reported risk in men who drank at least one daily diet soda, making them more prone to multiple myeloma and non-Hodgkin's lymphoma than non- diet-soda drinkers.

Active Agents: Common artificial sweeteners are sucralose, aspartame, saccharin, Equal, NutraSweet, Stevia, Sugar Twin, Sweet "N Low, Splenda, etc. Newer is erythritol, associated with increased blood clotting and a two-fold higher risk for heart attack and stroke.

Essential Advice: *Don't substitute diet sodas for sugary sodas, assuming they are okay or better when in truth they are far worse. Avoid diet sodas and drink more water, milk, and lower calorie juices.*

DIETARY PATTERNS

Worst and Best Diets

Obviously, the foods you eat most often are most apt to determine how long you live. Four of the best recognized and tested dietary patterns in the United States are Prudent, Western, Traditional, and Fish and Alcohol. When applied to 13,466 Americans aged 18 to 90, during a twenty-year research study, here's how the dietary patterns fared in promoting longevity:

1. Only the "Prudent" diet improved longevity. It was linked to a 10 percent *lower* risk of overall death odds, although it did not reduce odds of fatal cancer. The diet is high in vegetables, fruits, and low in meat and oils.

2. The widespread "Western" diet, common in the US and Europe, is the most lethal. It *increased* overall death risk 22 percent and upped fatal cancer odds 33 percent. It is rich in sweets and oils and low in fruits and vegetables.

3. A "Traditional" diet *increased* death risk by 16 percent, and fatal cancer odds by 15 percent. It is high in red meat, eggs, legumes, potatoes, and bread.

4. A "Fish and Alcohol Diet" was *neutral,* not apt to reduce or increase risk of overall death or fatal cancer. It is high in fish, seafood and alcoholic beverages compared to other diets.

Among those in the "study group of Americans:" seven percent died of cerebrovascular disease, 22 percent of cancer, 24 percent of cardiovascular disease, and 48 percent of other causes.

Essential Advice: *Make your dietary pattern high in fruits and vegetables, and low in oils and meat. Among these four diets, go with the Prudent Diet and run away as fast as you can from the awful Western Diet.*

EATING DISORDERS

Skyrocketing Deaths

Eating disorders are on the rise, afflicting nine percent of the world's population, including twenty-nine million Americans, of whom 26 percent attempt suicide and 10,000 succeed yearly, often from self-starvation.

Two most common food disorders, anorexia nervosa and bulimia nervosa, increase the odds of dying by 500 percent! Two newer eating disorders-- binge eating disorder (BED) and avoidance/restrictive food intake disorder (ARFID) are also deadly.

Once confined to Western nations, anorexia and bulimia, have spread to Asian and Middle Eastern countries. Although traditionally considered female maladies, they also are thriving among adolescent men as well as young women. Males, however, are more prone to binge eating disorders.

The severity of eating disorders is also worsening, according to a 2020 survey. Here are their symptoms to be on guard against:

Anorexia Nervosa, characterized by significant weight loss, fear of gaining weight, and failure to recognize the severity of low body weight.

Bulimia Nervosa, characterized by binge eating, is defined as consuming a large amount of food within a two-hour period while experiencing a lack of control over what or how much one is consuming.

Binge-eating disorder is a new eating disorder of recurrent episodes of at least one binge episode each week for three months.

Avoidant /Restrictive Food Intake Disorder is a new diagnosis in which disruptions in eating compromise nutritional needs due to irrational reasons.

Essential Advice: *Look for eating disorders mainly in early to late adolescence. If suspected, take immediate action and get professional treatment. With treatment 60 percent recover from eating disorders; without, 20 percent die.*

EGGS

The Scare Factor is Back

Historically, a fear of eggs has focused on a cholesterol heart scare. Now the graver central issue is: can eggs trigger premature death, likely due to a link with chronic diseases, including cancer? A recent worldwide study of 50 countries concluded that eating ten eggs a week (about one and a half a day) accelerated overall death prospects by 13 percent.

In a 2019 bombshell study from Northwestern University, researchers tracked the egg consumption of nearly 30,000 middle-aged Americans for 17 years. The alarming discovery: adding only half a daily egg to your diet was associated with an eight percent surge in death rates. Worse, the higher the consumption of eggs, the higher the probability of death. Curiously, enthusiastic female egg-eaters had four times more fatal heart attacks than males.

The most surprising "nail in the coffin" came in 2021. A diet analysis of half a million elderly Americans concluded that eating a mere extra half an egg a day was potentially deadly. Further, researchers identified cholesterol in the yolk as the lethal agent. They blamed an extra 300 milligrams of cholesterol a day (the amount in two small egg yolks) for escalating death odds a remarkable 19 per cent, mainly due to cancer and cardiovascular disease.

The latest warning: In 2022 Harvard researchers noted that the highest egg consumers compared to the lowest, were *20 per cent more apt to die of cancer.*

Active Agents: Eggs' likely deadliest villain is high cholesterol in the egg yolk, say researchers.

Essential Advice: *Whether you eat eggs depends on how much risk you want to tolerate. Assuming the worst risk is in the egg yolk from the cholesterol, you could eat only egg whites. Otherwise, limiting eggs to none or fewer than three whole eggs per week makes longevity sense.*

EGGPLANT

Ancient Staple with Purple Power

Eggplant as medicine can be traced back 4,000 years to India where it was used to treat diabetes. Italians once called eggplant the "apple of madness," in the belief that eating it would drive you insane.

Scientists today hail eggplant as a large berry-vegetable with a bunch of recently discovered unique biochemical characteristics.

Eggplant's greatest claim to fame is a rare and powerful anthocyanin compound concentrated mostly in the pigment of the eggplant's dark purple skin. Most important, anthocyanins, rich in all deep red, blue and purple fruits, and vegetables, are endowed with remarkably strong antioxidant disease-fighting activity.

Among 120 vegetables, eggplant ranked in the top ten in antioxidant powers enabling it to defuse free radical chemicals, thus fighting off death and disease from countless infections and chronic diseases. Eggplant has been used notably in Asian and Middle

Eastern countries to treat asthma, bronchitis, arthritis, diabetes and high cholesterol.

Some experts call purple foods like eggplant with high concentrations of anthocyanins "superfoods," because they promote cardiovascular health, help prevent cancer and dementia and increase longevity. Eggplant also reportedly contains a molecule with potential therapeutic benefit against Alzheimer's disease.

Essential Advice: *Eat eggplant's purple skin, as well as flesh for its maximum longevity activity, as well as its antioxidant, anti-inflammatory, cardioprotective, anti-obesity, anti-diabetic, and anti-cancer properties. Don't grill or fry eggplant at high temperatures which depletes its antioxidant activity.*

FASTING

Controversial Way to Prolong Life

Taking regular breaks from eating is called fasting or "intermittent fasting." The idea, originating in the early twentieth century, relies on frequent interruptions to shorten the time you devote to eating, obviously reducing food intake and weight gain.

However, the main point of "intermittent fasting," authorities insist, is to trip a metabolic button, initiating cellular changes that discourage weight gain and fatal chronic diseases, while promoting longevity.

Extensive evidence finds that fasting can counter diabetes, cardiovascular disease, cancer, and prolong life in animals and humans. A 2023 University of Wisconsin study concluded that monkeys who ate 30 per cent fewer calories had half the death rates of monkeys that ate whatever they pleased. One "fasting" monkey died at age 44, the equivalent of 134 years for a human.

There is also a less stringent method of fasting, called the Fasting Mimicking Diet, that lasts five days and allows some calories, while still providing the benefits of a calorie-free fast. It was developed by Dr. Valter Longo, director of the Longevity Institute at the University of Southern California.

Nevertheless, the National Institute on Aging says no studies so far have produced evidence that fasting of any kind expands the lifespan of humans.

Essential Advice: *If you want to try any form of fasting for an extended time, such as weeks or months, consult your doctor or other medical professional to avoid inadvertently starving and harming yourself.*

FATS & OILS

The Best, Worse, and Just Awful

For advice on which fats and oils to eat, the likely answer used to be: "Fat is a four-letter word that should be banished from your diet." The current wisdom is: "Since various dietary fats drive death risks up or down, you must carefully choose which fats to eat or avoid."

Here's how five common fats and oils are likely to extend or shorten life, based mainly on three decades of Harvard research.

Omega-3 Fish Fats: Major research shows that lifesaving omega-3 fats in seafood (fatty fish and fish oil supplements) lower death odds by seven percent.

Monounsaturated Fats: Olive oil, avocado, canola, peanut, high oleic safflower and sunflower oils cut death odds by eleven per cent.

Omega-6 polyunsaturated vegetable fats: Corn, peanut, safflower, sunflower and soybean oils slash death risk by nineteen percent.

Saturated fats: Primarily animal fats. A major British study in 2020 found that reducing the intake of saturated fat had "little or no effect" on human deaths due to cardiovascular disease or any other cause.

Trans Fats: Decidedly the worst are man-made industrial trans fats. Banned in the United States, they accelerate death rates by thirteen percent. Also, to be avoided are *"partially hydrogenated oils,* the primary source of deadly trans fats.

Active Agents: Certain fats incite inflammation, clog arteries, stimulate weight gain, and mess up other biochemical processes.

Essential Advice: *Replace bad fats with better fats. Omega-3 fish fat is good. Polyunsaturated and monounsaturated fats, such as olive oil, are okay. Saturated animal fats are iffy. Man-made trans fats are abominable and should never touch your lips.*

FERMENTED FOOD

"Bad" Food for a Longer Life

The ancient Egyptians, Babylonians, and Chinese preserved foods by fermenting them or exposing them to live bacteria. Science now understands that consuming fermented food overrun by specific live bacteria, increases human resistance to an array of chronic inflammatory diseases that are the world's primary causes of death.

Thus, eating fermented foods promotes longevity by helping prevent diabetes, gastrointestinal disorders, cardiovascular disease, cancer, and obesity.

For example: fermenting cabbage transforms it into sauerkraut, tripling its longevity activity. The traditional Japanese diet, supporting one of the world's longest living populations, features fermented foods at virtually every meal, including pickles, miso (soybean paste), soy sauce, and kimchi (pickled vegetables).

A Swedish study of about a million people found that a mere two thirds of an ounce of daily yogurt with live bacterial cultures is likely to cut overall death rates by two percent.

Common fermented foods apt to increase longevity are kefir, probiotic yogurt, tempeh, natto, miso, soy sauce, kombucha tea, kimchi or sauerkraut, sourdough bread, pecorino cheese, table olives, and vinegar.

Active Agents: Fermentation, due to bacteria, creates anti-inflammatory and immunomodulatory activity.

Essential Advice: *Eat fermented foods every day or as often as you please, to help ward off chronic diseases. Food labels on fermented foods should say "contains probiotics or contains live cultures." Be aware that fermented foods may also be high in sodium.*

FIBER

King of Longevity

Eating high-fiber foods puts you on the fast track to longevity. Dozens of studies show death odds sink dramatically when you eat high-fiber whole grains, seeds, fruits and vegetables. Yet our modern diet is "fiber impoverished." Ninety five percent of Americans eat only half the 25 to 30 grams of daily food fiber recommended by the American Heart Association.

Overwhelming evidence of fiber 's power to deter death comes from a 2019 World Health Organization analysis of 240 studies. The highest-fiber eaters compared to the least lived the longest. Eating a mere extra eight grams of fiber daily, the amount in one cup of raspberries, slashed the risk of fatal heart disease and diabetes by five to 27 percent.

A large new ten-year Korean study showed that the likelihood of death doubled in those who skimped on fiber compared to those who ate foods packed with fiber. When Mediterranean diet advocates ate eight ounces of high-fiber fruit a day their chances of death dropped an astonishing 41 percent!

At least a dozen studies reveal that eating the most cereal fiber compared with the least, cuts overall death risk by 19 percent, cardiovascular disease by 18 percent and cancer by 15 percent. Interestingly, in Japan eating fiber in legumes, fruits and vegetables reduced mortality, but eating cereal fiber did not.

Active Agents: Fiber in foods, both water soluble and insoluble, have been shown to increase longevity.

Essential Advice: *Increase your intake of whole grains, high-fiber cereals, brown rice, legumes, fresh fruit including peels when appropriate, and vegetables raw and cooked. Check food labels. No other single nutritional element is more life-promoting than fiber.*

FISH

First Course for Aspiring Immortals

Fish is a sure bet to help avoid a premature collision with death, *but only if the fish is fatty*. The source of fish's longevity advantage are high levels of omega-3 fatty acids (EPA and DHA), that circulate throughout our blood and tissues after we eat fatty fish.

High concentrations of omega-3 fats in our bodies due to eating fatty fish predict a long life, and low levels of omega-3's due to skimping on fatty fish forecast a premature death. In a study of 42,000 men and women those with the highest blood levels of omega-3 fatty acids were 18 percent *less likely to die for any reason* than those low in blood omega-3s due to a low-fish diet.

Recent updated Italian research stresses that only "fatty" fish, not "lean" fish bestow longevity. "Fatty fish" are salmon, tuna, herring, kippers, mackerel, eel, trout and sardines. "Lean" fish are cod, plaice, shellfish, seabass, sole, tilapia, and orange roughy.

There is no evidence that eating *lean* fish provides any significant longevity benefits.

However, not to worry if you don't eat lots of fatty fish. Fish oil supplements are a spectacular substitute. In a study of 427,678 men and women, taking fish oil for 12 years cut overall death risk by 13 percent. In other research doses of fish oil cut cardiac deaths by 20 percent. And taking 850 milligrams of fish oil every day for three and a half years slashed chances of sudden cardiac death by 45 per cent.

Active Agents: The fatty acids in fish fight inflammation, lower blood pressure and regulate other processes in ways that encourage longevity.

Essential Advice: *Eat fatty fish at least three times or more a week and take fish oil supplements if needed. The typical routine average dose of fish oil is 1000 milligrams of omega-3s daily, and 4,000 milligrams daily to reduce high triglycerides.*

FLAVONOIDS

Life- Stretching Antioxidants

Plants are packed with mighty longevity phytochemicals called flavonoids. Foods with the most flavonoids are berries of all types, red cabbage, citrus fruits, cocoa and chocolate, kale, red and white onions, parsley, soybeans, tea, and red wine. All flavonoids have strong antioxidant activity, defusing free radical oxygen reactions that promote disease and aging.

Such flavonoids primarily protect the heart, blood vessels and brain. A recent major study of nearly 100,000 Americans, average age 70, revealed that those who ate the most flavonoids compared to the least were 18 percent less apt to die of cardiovascular disease.

In elderly men who splurged on flavonoid-rich foods the risk of fatal stroke dropped 37 percent! Remarkably, the amount of flavonoids needed to initiate the process of longevity is low—for example in one study an ounce and half of blueberries was sufficient to rev up significant longevity activity.

In other research, high flavonoids in cocoa and black tea exhibited strong powers to lower high blood pressure. Another study documented improved constriction and dilation of blood vessels after consumption of high-flavonoid cocoa, blueberries, black tea, cranberry juice, orange juice and apples.

Blood flow to the brain improved after drinking dark cocoa or blueberry juice. Some research finds that high-flavonoid foods and drinks help prevent age-related neurodegeneration.

Active Agents: Subclasses of flavonoids are also known as epicatechins in tea, anthocyanins in blueberries, red wine, and strawberries, and genistein in soybeans and peanuts.

Essential Advice: *Go wild. Eat as many flavonoid-rich foods as you want but beware of excessive alcohol in wine.*

FRIED FOODS

Everybody's Fatal Attraction

A recent 20-year study of 107,000 late middle-aged women by University of Iowa scientists concluded that eating fried food every day, compared to none, raised odds of premature death an average eight percent. Specifically, eating fried chicken, fried fish, or shellfish once a week boosted early death odds by 12 to 13 percent. A daily dose of fried chicken increased the risk of death from cardiovascular disease by 23 percent.

Not surprisingly, the more daily servings of fried foods the women ate, the greater their risk of death increased.

Deep fried foods appear more dangerous than pan-fried. In certain studies eating deep fried foods more than twice a week, compared with once a week, raised the risk of certain cancers, particularly of the stomach, gallbladder, prostrate and pancreas by as much as one third.

In other research Harvard investigators have reported that eating fried foods every day boosted the risk of developing type 2 diabetes in both women and men by 55 percent.

When public health officials in China looked at the dangers of fried food, they found that citizens who ate the most compared with the least were 16 percent more likely to be overweight, 20 percent more apt to have high blood pressure and 37 per cent more apt to have a stroke or heart failure.

Active Agents: The most commonly blamed villain in fried foods are trans fatty acids created by high temperatures. Other culprits: salt and life-threatening byproducts such as advanced glycation end products (ages) and acrylamide, notably in French fries.

Essential Advice: *Avoid or cut down on all fried foods, especially deep-fried chicken, fish, and French fries, as well as potato chips and donuts.*

FRUITS & VEGETABLES

Longevity Super Stars

The toll for ignoring fruits and vegetables is staggering. Experts blame a fruit and vegetable "deficiency" for 5.6 to 7.8 million premature deaths worldwide every year, mainly from heart disease, strokes, and cancer.

Dozens of studies hail fruits and vegetables as a passport to longevity. For decades standard advice was to eat seven fruits and vegetables a day. Then in 2021 Harvard researchers declared five a day (two fruits and three vegetables) "optimal," based on data showing that five fruits and vegetables per day cut death odds 13 percent among two million adults. Eating more than five did not further increase longevity. Sadly, Americans average only one and a half fruits and vegetables a day.

Most potent in stifling cardiac and stroke deaths in many studies are juices, garlic, citrus, grapes, and carrots. Research also reveals a steep fall in death odds with increased intakes of apples, pears, citrus fruits, green leafy vegetables, cruciferous vegetables, and salads.

Raisins, prunes, dates, figs, cranberries, apricots and other dried fruits are more powerfully anti-death than raw fruit. In one study eating dried fruit three to five times a week cut fatal pancreatic cancer odds by 65 percent!

Raw vegetables are more powerful in extending life than cooked. Some experts advise eating at least half of your vegetables raw. Choose bright colored fruits and vegetables; pigment is an antioxidant.

Active Agents: Fruits and vegetables contain an array of antioxidants and other life boosting chemicals.

Essential Advice: *Eat at least five fruits and vegetables daily, including the peel when appropriate. It often contains most of a fruit's antioxidant clout, for example, apple peels. Don't let these powerful outer parts of a fruit or vegetable go to waste.*

GARLIC

The Grandee of Lifesaving Herbs

Garlic was found in Egyptian pyramids and Greek temples and prescribed in ancient Italian and Chinese medical textbooks. Modern science verifies garlic's anti-aging powers to inhibit various cancers, reduce the risk of cardiovascular disease and stroke, and boost intellectual functioning as well as longevity.

The best evidence comes from a study of 27,000 men and women over age 80 living in China, where garlic is revered and widely consumed. That's where investigators at UCLA and the University of Pennsylvania went to learn about garlic's strong connection with longevity.

They asked elderly Chinese participants: How often do you eat garlic now and when you were age 60? A choice of answers: *"often"* (more than five times a week), *"occasionally"* (one to four times a week) or *"rarely"* (less than once a week.)

After 13 years of study, the researchers came to this striking conclusion: "Without a doubt, the oldest old who ate garlic most often survived longest. " The death risk of those who ate garlic more than five times a week was 11 percent lower than that of those who ate garlic less than once a week. The five-times-a week garlic eaters also were less likely to have hypertension, cognitive impairment, and other aging-related diseases than the infrequent garlic eaters.

Active Agents: Garlic is packed with various antioxidants called organosulfur compounds which are credited for its superior longevity benefits.

Essential Advice: *Eat garlic "often" or five times a week--preferably raw, which is how the Chinese usually consume it, to get the highest concentration of longevity- provoking antioxidants.*

GLYCEMIC RATING

Major Clue to Longevity

All foods have a so-called glycemic index, a number revealing how high and rapidly they cause blood sugar to spike after digestion. The glycemic index is widely hailed as a measure of each food's impact on longevity.

A diet full of sugary foods with a high-glycemic index forecasts a shorter life. And a diet of foods less apt to spike blood sugar predicts a longer life.

In a twenty-country study of about 138,000 individuals ages 35 to 70, those who ate the highest glycemic index diets, compared to the lowest, were 25 to 50 percent more apt to die of any cause, particularly of cardiovascular disease.

Each person's diet was analyzed, based on how high each food caused blood sugar to surge after ingestion. For example, foods might have the following glycemic indexes: dairy, 38; legumes, 42; non-starchy vegetables, 54; fruit juice, 68; fruit, 69; white bread, 100. Each participant's diet was then assigned an average glycemic index. The subjects were tracked for a decade.

The conclusion documented that eating foods with a high glycemic index are far more likely to cause higher overall death rates and cardiovascular deaths than diets with a low glycemic index.

Here is a rough guide to the glycemic index of foods: *High:* white rice, white bread, white potatoes, crackers, doughnuts, cold breakfast cereals, sugary desserts. *Medium:* corn, bananas, raisins, whole grain cereals. *Low:* most fruits and vegetables, legumes, beans, peas, lentils, pasta, low fat dairy foods, nuts.

Essential Advice: *Eat foods with a lower glycemic index. Avoid or restrict foods with a high glycemic index. Check online for charts showing the glycemic index and glycemic load of all common foods.*

GRAPES & RAISINS

Resveratrol May Slow Aging

Grapes and raisins were a cure for old age in ancient Persia and Greece, and still may have a huge future. With the worldwide explosion of people over age 60 about to grow by two billion during the next half century, so does the demand for anti-aging foods. High on the scientific agenda are foods bursting with a longevity chemical called resveratrol. The major sources are grape skin, grape juice and dried grapes known as raisins.

Research suggests that resveratrol may help protect against cardiovascular diseases, sarcopenia, cancers, osteoporosis, and neurodegenerative diseases, such as Alzheimer's.

In animals, resveratrol has increased the production of neurons and improved memory, learning, and mood. It also delayed the aging process related to cardiovascular disease by reducing inflammation, discouraging formation of blood clots and lowering bad LDL cholesterol. Many studies show that resveratrol increases muscle mass, strength and endurance and bone growth. It also helps fight off the invasion and spread of cancerous tumors.

Several clinical trials reveal resveratrol's anti-aging effects in humans. For example, eating 200 milligrams a day of resveratrol improved memory in older adults. In a sixteen-year British study of 30,000 women, those who ate at least three ounces of fresh grapes per day compared to none were 34 percent less likely to have fatal cardiovascular disease!

Essential Advice: *Eat foods rich in resveratrol including grapes, raisins, peanuts, blueberries, cucumbers, tomatoes, red cabbage, and spinach. Okay also is red wine in moderation. High doses of isolated resveratrol taken as a supplement are controversial, and generally not recommended by nutritional authorities to thwart aging.*

GREEN LEAFY VEGETABLES

Essential for Longevity

If there were such a thing as a "Methusela Meter," to measure a food's innate powers to extend life, green leafy vegetables would rank number one in the universe. No food generates stronger longevity activity than leafy greens, including spinach, kale, leaf lettuce, arugula, beet greens, watercress, romaine lettuce, swiss chard, bok choy, and turnip greens.

Extensive evidence shows that leafy greens are strongly intertwined with longevity. Harvard investigators detected only one third as much fatal cancer in people who ate the most green vegetables, compared to the least. A 2020 study in the *Journal of the American Heart Association* linked eating a single daily serving of leafy greens with an 18 percent drop in fatal cardiovascular disease.

A 2021 Japanese analysis of 24 studies showed that three and a half ounces of leafy greens a day was tied to a 25 percent drop in overall death odds. Yet only about 10 percent of Americans eat the recommended quota of vegetables, including leafy greens.

In far-out research, University of Alabama scientists even discovered that leafy greens are an antidote to colon-cancer-promoting foods such as red meat. In a test, fifty obese adults ate red meat ten times a week, along with a daily half cup of cooked spinach, kale, collards or turnip greens.

After researchers doubled the greens to a full daily cup for three months, they were astonished to note profound changes in the subjects' intestinal tracts that created a biochemical barrier, blocking colon cancer's progression to become deadly. They concluded that the increased life-promoting anti-cancer activity was due to the extra daily half cup of greens!

Essential Advice: *It's not just smart but essential for anyone who wants to live the longest life possible to eat green leafy vegetables every day, at least half a cup or more, raw or cooked.*

HERBS & SPICES

Tiny Doses Extend Survival

Dozens of herbs and spices, used in tiny amounts to flavor food, flood our bodies with antioxidants and other longevity chemicals. Number one in antioxidant potency on a list of 425 dried and ground spices and herbs is clove, followed by peppermint, allspice, cinnamon, oregano, thyme, sage, rosemary, and saffron.

A major study by the National Cancer Institute tracked 50,045 participants over an 11-year-period, to find out whether herb usage delayed death. They documented that turmeric consumption is associated with a reduced ten percent overall death risk; black pepper with eight percent lower death odds; saffron with a 15 percent lower risk of overall death and a 19 percent drop in risk of fatal cardiovascular disease.

Recent lab and clinical studies also reveal multiple life-promoting activities of herbs and spices. Cinnamon thwarts the metastatic spread of cancer, lowers blood pressure and has anti-inflammatory activity. Ginger markedly lowers cholesterol and triglycerides. Black pepper has remarkable antioxidant and anti-inflammatory effects.

A low dose of turmeric decreased blood cholesterol by 12 percent and increased HDL good cholesterol by 29 percent. Fenugreek seeds helped prevent alcohol-induced liver damage. The herb rosemary improved vascular function and reduced diabetic complications. Death risk from cardiovascular disease fell 17 per cent in regular consumers of ginseng.

Active Agents: Various herbs and spices contribute a multitude of phytochemicals that deliver tiny boosts of longevity.

Essential Advice: *Liberally use common herbs and spices to add an unknown amount of time to your life span.*

HONEY & MAPLE SYRUP

Super Sugar Busters

Which sweetener would you identify as a longevity superstar: honey, maple syrup or sugar? Science declares both honey and maple syrup far superior to sugar. A study at the University of Wales, for example, showed that a group of men who reported eating honey over a 25-year period had death odds 56 percent lower than men who said they didn't eat honey.

Honey is an ancient folk medicine with antibacterial, antioxidant, antitumor, and antiviral activity. It revs up immune functioning and anti-inflammatory activity, supposedly explaining its ability to thwart various cancers and reduce negative effects from cancer drugs. Its powers are attributed to a resinous substance produced by honeybees called propolis. New Japanese research suggests honey also helps prevent covid 19.

A modern scientific appraisal of maple syrup reveals strong antiproliferative, antimicrobial, and exceptionally high antioxidant and anti-cancer properties. University of Rhode Island pharmacists recently discovered thirty previously unknown biologically active phytochemicals in maple syrup.

Dark-colored maple syrup is credited with drug-like powers to block the proliferation, migration, and invasion of deadly pancreatic cancer cells. Other research identifies maple syrup constituents that help protect against type-2 diabetes.

Active Agents: The main phytochemical in honey is called propolis and maple syrup contains various chemical phenolics, vitamins and minerals.

Essential Advice: *Substitute both honey and maple syrup as unique natural sweeteners for ordinary common sugars and artificial sweeteners.*

ICE CREAM

Cool Way to Flirt with Death

The worst sign that ice cream may *not* be good for you: it is officially categorized as an "ultra-processed food," ranked at the bottom of the heap among authorities on health, diet and longevity. Research says eating ultra-processed foods more than four times a day raises death odds an astounding sixty two percent! Further, each additional serving raises death expectations 18 percent. Such foods also increase your risk of obesity, cardiovascular disease, and cancer.

Ice cream typically is high in calories and added sugar and low in nutrients even when it's categorized as low-fat, and no-sugar added.

A 2023 British study reported that every ten per cent intake increase in such ultra-processed foods raises overall cancer risk by two percent, and ovarian cancer risk by 19 percent. Researchers at Kaiser Permanente in California showed that women with breast cancer who ate high-fat dairy foods, including ice cream, just once a day, were 64 percent more likely to die over the next 12 years. Possible culprit, according to researchers: high estrogen in ice cream's major ingredient milk, and a potential trigger of tumor growth.

The good news: there is some minor conflicting evidence. A recent study found a 38 percent lower risk of endometriosis in women who ate ice cream once or more a day as adolescents than those who ate less ice cream. Also, a team of stellar academics declared that eating ice cream might slightly reduce the risk of pancreatic cancer, although forthcoming evidence is needed to verify it.

Essential Advice: *While we wait for more direct conclusive evidence, it is wise to think of ice cream as an occasional treat, not a daily indulgence. Also be sure to choose lower-sugar, lower-fat, lower-calorie brands of ice cream.*

THE JAPANESE DIET

Adds Years to Your Earth Time

Japan holds a world record for longevity. In 2022 life expectancy in Japan was 88.09 years for females and 81.91 for males, the highest among 193 countries. In sharp contrast, the United States ranks 46th in the world with a life expectancy of 81.65 years for females and 76.61 for males. A typical Japanese man lives about five years longer and a Japanese woman seven years longer than American men and women.

Scientists theorize that much of the extraordinary Japanese longevity is tied to their unique diet.

Although the Japanese diet has become more Westernized lately, it traditionally includes daily portions of rice, miso soup, soybean products, vegetables, fruits, fish, Japanese pickles, seaweed, mushrooms, and green tea. Sweets and meat are less common. Fermented foods are more common.

A recent analysis of 90,000 Japanese adults revealed that those who strongly embrace Japan's traditional diet compared to those who don't, are 14 percent less apt to die for any reason and 11 percent less apt to succumb to fatal cardiovascular disease. Devotees of the Japanese diet are also six percent less apt to die from cancer and 11 percent less apt to die from cerebrovascular disease.

As for individual foods, eating seaweed and green and yellow vegetables predicts a six percent lower death risk. Death risk also drops five percent due to eating pickles, three percent due to fish and 11 percent for green tea. Not surprisingly, eating beef and pork appears to *increase* death odds by two percent.

Essential Advice: *As expected, the Japanese Diet encourages life, discourages death and is a life-prolonging protocol to follow.*

JUICES

Not the Super Food You Think

Don't count on fruit and vegetable juices to help you live longer. On the other hand, there is alarming evidence that drinking juices threatens longevity, shortening rather than expanding life.

That unexpected message emerged loud and clear from a 2022 government study of 40,000 Americans who said they drank a daily cup or more of 100 percent fruit juice over a ten-year period. Indeed, those who did so faced this grim fact: Drinking eight ounces or more of fruit juice a day was associated with a 30 per cent jump in overall death odds and a 49 percent rise in fatal heart disease risk, compared with drinking no juice!

Another analysis of 30,000 American men and women reported a 24 percent *increased* risk of death for each additional 12 ounces of 100 percent juice consumed.

Harvard researchers also found that drinking fruit juice every day is likely to increase blood glucose and insulin and your risk of diabetes by 21 percent.

A possible reason: Juices are typically stripped of fiber, and higher in sugar and sodium compared with whole fruits and vegetables. One nutrition expert calls commercial juices "high calorie sugar water."

Tests by Consumer Reports in 2019 found that 21 out of 45 commercial juices contained high levels of heavy metals potentially harmful to children.

Disturbing bottom line: juices do not equal whole fruits and vegetables as promoters of longevity.

Essential Advice: *Many experts say it's ok for adults to drink six ounces of fruit juice and eight ounces of vegetable juice a day. The American Academy of Pediatrics recommends the following daily juice limits for children: none if under age one, four ounces up to age three, six ounces up to age six and eight ounces after age seven.*

KALE

God's Gift to Longevity

When Hippocrates, the ancient Greek physician, said " Let food be thy medicine and medicine be thy food," he was describing what we now call "functional foods," or in modern lingo "superfoods." No food better fits that image than a dark green curly leafy vegetable known as kale. Its popularity has soared in the last decade as one of the superstars of the Mediterranean Diet.

Tests show that kale is blessed with a broad spectrum of strong antioxidant and anti-cancer activity. In fact, kale surpasses other high-powered vegetables in the brassica clan, such as broccoli, Brussels sprouts, and cauliflower, for high antioxidant activity. Kale also suppresses the proliferation of cancer cells, and has strong anti-inflammatory, anti-ulcer, and antimicrobial activity.

In men with high blood cholesterol, drinking five fluid ounces of kale juice per day for twelve weeks improved their HDL and LDL cholesterol and reduced inflammation, a major promoter of cardiovascular disease and premature death.

Kale is the most prominent star in the Brassica plant species. It floods our bodies with unique flavonoids whose mission is to thwart cardiovascular disease, cancer, diabetes, Alzheimer's disease, cataracts, and age-related functional decline.

Active Agents: Kale is particularly rich in anti-cancer isothiocyanates found to primarily reduce the risk of kidney, prostate, colorectal cancers, as well as lung, breast and oral cancers to a lesser degree.

Essential Advice: *Don't ignore kale; it is a powerful longevity ally. Store it in the refrigerator and use it immediately after chopping to minimize loss of its longevity powers due to its carotenoids and flavonoids.*

KETO DIET

Controversial and Risky

About 13 million Americans (five percent) follow a very low- carbohydrate high-fat diet ranked at the bottom of acceptable diets by leading nutritionists. Called the *ketogenic or keto diet*, it severely restricts all carbohydrates--breads, grains, cereals, fruits and vegetables, beans and yogurt, usually considered pillars of good health. The diet favors excesses of fatty meat, butter, bacon and other parcels of potential harm.

The keto diet that originated in the 1920's to treat epilepsy in children is controversial and risky. In 2022 it was ranked the *worst* diet of the year by US News & World Report media organization, and at the bottom of the heap again in 2023.

Medical experts link the keto diet to a greater risk of cardiovascular disease, low blood pressure, bad breath, kidney stones, constipation, nutrient deficiencies, menstrual irregularities and eating disorders. It also may lead to "keto flu" with symptoms of upset stomach, dizziness, mood swings and low energy.

The keto diet promotes weight loss by slashing carb intake to 10 percent of calories and exploding fat intake to 75 percent of calories. Unlike less strict low-carb diets, this creates ketosis, a period akin to famine, causing your body to burn ketones from fat instead of sugar from carbohydrates.

The critical difference: A standard diet is 45 to 65 percent carbs and 20-35 percent fat. A low carb diet is 30-40 percent carbs and 30 percent fat. A keto diet is a mere 5-10 percent carbs and 70-75 percent fat.

Essential Advice: *The super low-carb keto diet is touted to lead to fast weight loss, and may be a short-term success for some, but causes long-term problems for others. The diet has numerous harsh critics so only try it with trepidation at your own risk.*

MEAT CURED
Bacon, Ham, Hot Dogs, etc.

Ferocious Carcinogens

Eating more than five strips (five ounces) of bacon a week speeds up death's arrival--by eight percent from heart disease, stroke, and cancer; by nine percent from Alzheimer's; 12 percent from diabetes; 19 percent from kidney disease; 21 percent from respiratory diseases, and 22 percent from liver disease.

Meat is hazardous on its own, but curing it *doubles* its likelihood of killing you. Ordinarily eating an extra 3.5 ounces of red meat raises death risk nine percent. But if meat is "cured," with preservative chemicals, its odds of killing you soar to 17 percent. The odds of death from cardiovascular death jump to 19 percent, and from neurogenerative disease to 57 percent!

So deadly is cured meat that the World Health Organization bluntly calls it a class 1 carcinogen. In 2015 WHO announced that the *"existing evidence is sufficient to officially classify cured meat as a human carcinogen!"*

With every extra ounce of bacon, ham, bologna, or other cured meat you eat per day, your risk of death from cancer rises 20 percent, accounting for 14,500 new American deaths yearly. Another 58,000 Americans die annually from other cancers, heart disease, stroke, and type 2 diabetes linked to cured or "processed" meat. Eating one hot dog can shorten your life by 36 minutes, according to one report.

Active Agents: Curing meat with sodium, potassium nitrite or nitrate generates deadly carcinogenic poisons called nitrosamines and other chemicals within the meat and in your digestive tract.

Essential advice*: Avoid cured meats, including bacon, ham, hot dogs, salami, pastrami, bologna, pepperoni, kielbasa, corned beef, and all meat labeled as containing sodium nitrite or nitrate preservatives.*

MEAT UNCURED
Beef, Lamb, Pork, Veal

Powerful Assassins

A massive 16-year study of 536,969 Americans ages 50 to 71 by the National Cancer Institute showed that the more red meat you consume, the more likely you are to die--of most anything. Overall death rates in people who ate the most red meat, compared with the least, shot up 26 percent!

Specifically, among the highest red meat consumers, death odds from stroke soared 17 percent, from cancer 18 percent, from infections, 24 percent, from heart disease 27 percent, diabetes, 44 percent, kidney disease, 47 percent, respiratory diseases, 83 percent, and liver disease 130 percent.

Even a trifling amount of red meat—*less than two ounces a day*—boosted death odds ten percent among 81,000 U.S. health professionals in recent Harvard research. Red meat eaters who actually *increased* their intake over eight years by half a serving a day saw their death risk jump 20 percent over the next four years.

Particularly disturbing, a large Asian study noted that as red meat intake went up or down so did deaths from stroke. High meat intake is also associated with high rates of pancreatic cancer.

Active Agents: Red meat's major agent of destruction is reputedly heme iron, found only in animal flesh. (non heme iron occurs in plants). Overall deaths in the National Cancer Institute study jumped 15 percent in people getting the most heme iron from red meat.

Essential Advice: Eliminate or cut back on red meat. Restrict high heat frying and barbequing. Stewing, roasting and microwaving reduces, but does not eliminate red meat's deadly hazards.

MEDITERRANEAN DIET

World-Famous Diet

In the 1960's scientists discovered that populations in countries bordering the Mediterranean Sea lived longer with less chronic disease, due to eating a so-called "Mediterranean Diet." It became known as the world's number one most healthful diet, widely endorsed by authorities and research.

In a major analysis of 5200 individuals over age 65, those who strictly followed a Mediterranean diet for eight years cut their risk of death from any cause by *an astounding 25 percent*. A 2023 study of 700,000 American and European women showed that those eating a Mediterranean diet had 23 percent lower overall death rates. The National Institutes of Health estimates that the Mediterranean diet could reduce death rates about twenty percent in American men and women.

The earlier you begin a Mediterranean diet, the further your death prospects fall. Starting the diet at age 20 can add a decade to your life. Even starting at age

80 typically adds 3.4 years of life expectancy for both men and women.

The diet calls for a high consumption of fruits, nuts, vegetables, legumes, fish, whole grain cereals, olive oil and low consumption of all meats and dairy products, plus the option of a small glass of wine with food.

Active Agents: The diet is strongly anti-inflammatory, anti-cancer, lipid lowering, antimicrobial, and packed with antioxidants due to a variety of plant foods, and a little wine.

Essential Advice: *Go crazy for fruits, nuts, vegetables, legumes, fish, olive oil, and whole grains. Skimp on all meats and dairy products. Okay, or not: four to six ounces of red wine daily with food.*

THE MEDITERRANEAN "GREEN" DIET

Beyond Classic

In 2020 Harvard researcher Meir Stampfer decided to improve the Mediterranean Diet by adding leafy greens, rich in antioxidants. He also added three to four cups of green tea, an ounce of walnuts per day, and a few extra vegetables of your choice. Especially desirable, he said, was a tiny exotic plant called Mankai or duckweed, sold as a plant-based protein powder.

The new combination is called The Mediterranean "Green" Diet bolstered by a longer list of agreeable foods, including green tea, Mankai or duckweed, broccoli, green beans, cauliflower and onions, leafy greens, tomatoes, fruit, eggs, cottage cheese, yogurt, almonds, walnuts, olive oil, tahini, herbs, spices, small amounts of fish and poultry.

Still on the Mediterranean diet's negative list are red meat, processed or cured meat, highly processed foods like chips crackers and cereals, desserts, soda and other sweetened beverages.

Certain researchers declared "the Mediterranean Green Diet" superior to the original diet. Reportedly, eaters of the Med Green Diet compared with those on the regular Mediterranean Diet, have smaller waist circumferences, greater improvements in cholesterol, reductions in blood pressure and inflammatory activity, and higher cardiovascular scores.

Essential Advice: *You may get extra longevity benefits by adding greens and Mankai to the already superior Mediterranean Diet.*

MILK

How Much is Harmful?

Americans drink half as much milk today as in 1975--down from 29 gallons per capita to 16 gallons in 2021. Professor Karl Michaelsson at Uppsala University in Sweden says that's good for longevity.

Many scientists think likewise, although the evidence is somewhat in limbo. A recent three-decade study of 217,755 American health professionals concluded that 4.2 daily glasses of milk or servings of dairy foods, compared to three-fourths of a serving, hiked death rates seven percent. The likely villain: fat in milk.

That makes "whole" milk particularly worrisome. Recent research blamed a mere extra half cup of whole milk a day for spiking a 14 percent rise in overall death risk, including a 15 percent jump in risk of fatal cardiovascular disease and a 17 percent rise in deadly cancer odds.

Also important: skim (no fat) and low-fat milk do not significantly increase death rates. Weak evidence also links milk to prostate and ovarian cancer.

Then there's a scientific contingent that claims milk can *extend* life. One example: a 2023 twelve-year study of half a million women in the United Kingdom concluded that those consuming no-fat skim milk, semi-skimmed or soy milk had 18 *percent lower death rates than women drinking regular whole or fatty milk!*

On a final note, several large international studies reveal no significant connection between milk consumption and mortality.

Active Agents: whole milk is high in saturated fat that may promote inflammation and premature death.

Essential Advice: *Despite contradictions, many experts advise everyone after age two, including children, to shift to lower fat dairy and or restrict whole milk and, if desired, substitute soy milk, rice milk, oat milk, almond milk, and unflavored Greek yogurt. Choose organic milk to avoid antibiotics and hormones.*

MIND DIET

Puts Death on Dramatic Hold

Combine the Mediterranean Diet with the DASH Diet, and you get the Mind Diet, created in 2015 by Martha Clare Morris at Rush University Medical Center. She concluded that over-age-70 subjects who best complied with the Mind Diet for twelve years had *a remarkable 37 percent lower risk of premature death than the least compliant.*

MIND means Mediterranean-Dash Intervention for Neurodegenerative Delay. The diet reportedly lowers the risk of age-related cognitive decline and Alzheimer's disease and is remarkably easy to follow.

The diet calls for eating ten "healthy" foods (green leafy vegetables, other vegetables, nuts, berries, beans, whole grains, seafood, poultry, olive oil and wine) and avoiding five "unhealthy" foods (red meats, butter and stick margarine, cheese, pastries and sweets, and fried/fast food.)

Here are the commandments of the MIND Diet:

Eat at least three servings of whole grains a day.

Eat a salad every day.
Eat one other vegetable every day.
Snack almost daily on nuts.
Eat beans every other day.
Eat poultry and berries at least twice a week.
Eat fatty fish like salmon at least once a week.
Eat less than one tablespoon of butter per day.
Eat "unhealthy" food less than once a week.

Active Agents*: countless life-extending chemicals in the varied high antioxidant diet.*

Essential Advice: *Some authorities rate the Mind Diet superior to the Mediterranean Diet in longevity activity. It's well regarded among nutritional experts and well worth following.*

MUSHROOM

Behold the "Longevity Vitamin"

Mushrooms are a member of the stodgy fungal kingdom, and a "forgotten source of nutrients" for many people. Now thanks to Penn State College of Medicine researchers, mushrooms have emerged as the richest food source of a new super longevity entity they have christened "a longevity vitamin."

Penn State professor Djibril M. Ba PhD discovered that a diet rich in mushrooms parallels a drop in cancer risk after he scrutinized medical reports in Eastern Asian countries where consumption of mushrooms is exceptionally high. Specifically, he reported that a high mushroom intake of two-thirds of an ounce a day predicted a 45 percent drop in cancer risk, primarily breast cancer.

Moreover, he and colleagues isolated a unique antioxidant called ergothioneine, highly concentrated in shiitake, oyster, maitake and king oyster mushrooms which are widely consumed in East Asian countries.

White button, cremini and portobello mushrooms are more popular in the United States.

Dr. Ba credits the newly discovered mushroom antioxidant with far more than fighting off cancer. He says it discourages death from all causes. In 2021 Dr. Ba's massive meta-analysis with 601,893 individuals documented that eating modest amounts of any type mushroom is associated with at least a six percent drop-in overall death rates. Presumed to be the unique chemical responsible, ergothioneine was nicknamed "the longevity vitamin."

Active Agent: a powerful antioxidant called ergothioneine or "longevity vitamin."

Essential Advice: *Eat more mushrooms, especially shiitake, oyster, maitake and king oyster to boost your intake of mushrooms' so-called longevity vitamin.*

NUTS

Astonishing Morsels of Longevity

In a study of a million British, US and Norwegian subjects, those who ate a daily handful of any type nut were 22 percent less apt to die of any cause. Specifically, a few nuts every day lowered death odds by 35 percent from neurodegenerative disease, 39 percent from diabetes, 52 percent from respiratory diseases, 62 percent from kidney disease and 75 percent from infectious diseases.

Other research shows that eating a single ounce of walnuts, almonds, or hazelnuts every day for five years lowered risk of fatal cardiovascular events by 30 percent and of stroke in particular by 45 percent.

The toll from not eating nuts is staggering. Experts writing in a medical journal estimated that four and a half million people worldwide died prematurely in the year 2013 because they failed to eat a daily quota of nuts.

The optimal daily dose of nuts against premature death is 20 grams, a mere three quarters of an ounce, research suggests. Whether eating more can further prolong life is uncertain, although there is no reason to believe it would be detrimental in any way. Also eating peanut butter for unknown reasons did not lower death risk in a large National Institutes of Health study.

Active Agents: Fiber, vitamins, minerals, and various antioxidants that discourage multiple diseases and premature death.

Essential Advice: *No question, nuts are a powerful longevity superfood. Eat a handful or more every single day or 20 grams worth, which would consist of either 17 almonds, 13 cashews, 11 pecan halves, 10 English walnut halves, 8 hazelnuts, 6 Brazil nuts, or 25 peanuts. Of course, you can eat a combination.*

OATS

Superstar for All Time

The spectacular thing about oats: they are *whole grain*, with all the longevity powers that implies. Whether it's steel-cut oats, ordinary rolled oats, oat groats or instant oats--at its core, oatmeal is simply a marvel, always labeled "whole grain oats".

As expected, oats live up to grand expectations. An international study of 471,157 men and women by the University of Bern in 2021 showed that people who ate the most oatmeal compared to the least were 22 percent less apt to have diabetes, 19 percent less likely to have coronary heart disease and 21 per cent less apt to have a stroke.

Most striking: men and women who averaged roughly three-quarters of an ounce of oats a day had 26 percent lower odds of death from any cause.

A 2015 Harvard University study of 100,000 people similarly revealed that eating whole grains, equivalent to a small bowl of oatmeal, cut overall death risk by nine percent and heart disease death risk by 15 per cent compared to eating virtually no oats or whole grains.

According to the Centers for Disease Control and Prevention, eating oats makes you feel fuller, prevents constipation, improves blood cholesterol dramatically, lessens blood inflammation, regulates blood sugar and insulin levels, reduces cancer odds, and postpones your death.

Active Agents*:* Fiber is oats' secret weapon; three fourths of a cup of dry oats has three grams of soluble fiber.

Essential Advice: *For a significant longevity boost, eat at least half a cup of dry oats a day, prepared any way you like. More is quite unlikely to be harmful and likely to extend life further.*

OBESITY

The Truth About Death and Fat

True, being fat is not the best longevity booster. But neither does dropping pounds always scare death away.

A massive review by the Centers for Disease Control and Prevention of nearly 100 studies involving three million Americans documented that obesity, from mild to severe, escalates your likelihood of death by 18 percent. Among the severely obese, with a body mass index (BMI) of over 40, death risk soared 29 percent compared with being normal weight. In another study obese Danish men typically died eight years earlier than their normal-weight compatriots.

An especially intriguing finding: people who were overweight, but not obese, actually had six percent *lowe*r chances of death in some research.

And oddly, weight fluctuations are a major villain in premature deaths. One study revealed that death odds doubled after severe weight loss, whereas severe weight *gain* spiked death rates 23 percent. In fact, extensive evidence suggests that weight *loss* tends to jibe with rising death rates more than *gaining* weight does. However, the most important scientific takeaway stresses that the least apt to die are people who maintain a steady stable weight, without dramatic ups and downs.

Active Agents: Too much fat accumulation corrupts normal bodily processes, but so do weight loss and fluctuations.

Essential Advice: *Avoid severe weight variations and try to maintain a stable normal BMI of 18.5 to under 25. To calculate your BMI: multiply your weight in pounds by 703, then divide by your height in inches once, then divide again.*

OLIVE OIL

Best Oil for a Long Life

Olive oil is extraordinarily potent in extending your stay on earth. Among 40,000 people in Spain, (the world's top producer of olive oil), those who ate the most olive oil compared with none, were 26 percent less apt to die of any cause and 44 percent less likely to die of cardiovascular disease during a thirteen-year-long study.

According to a new American study of 60,582 women and 31,801 men, eating a mere half a tablespoon of olive oil a day compared to rarely eating olive oil was related to a 19 percent plunge in overall death risk during 28 months. The committed olive oil consumers also reported seven percent lower odds of fatal cancer, 29 per cent lower odds of deadly neurogenerative disease, and 18 percent lower risk of fatal respiratory disease.

Additional evidence shows that olive oil helps prevent heart attacks, and cancer of the upper aerodigestive tract, breast and possibly colon. Women who ate more than one tablespoon of olive oil a day were ten percent less apt to develop type 2 diabetes.

Substituting olive oil for equal amounts of margarine, butter, mayonnaise and dairy fat appeared to precipitate an eight percent drop in overall death risk.

Active Agents: Scientists credit olive oil's high monounsaturated fatty acids and antioxidant polyphenols for its longevity benefits, which are much higher in extra virgin olive oil than in ordinary olive oil.

Essential Advice: *Use extra virgin olive oil which tests superior to regular olive oil in cutting the risk of fatal heart disease. Eat at least a tablespoon a day of extra virgin olive oil, experts advise.*

ONION

A Star but Not Quite a Superstar

For centuries onions have been worshiped by ancient Egyptians and devoured by Greek and Phoenician sailors to prevent scurvy. Worldwide 170 countries produce 78 million tons of onions annually. The average American eats 35 pounds of onions a year.

Onion's life-promoting talents are substantial but not legendary. All onions (red, violet, white and green) possess multiple phytochemicals that are antimicrobial, antioxidant, analgesic, anti-inflammatory, antidiabetic, anti-hypertensive, and anti-cancer. Particularly life-promoting is quercetin, an antioxidant disease-fighting flavonoid. Onions have five to ten times more quercetin than broccoli, apples, or blueberries.

This means that onions can zap microbes responsible for causing infections, including *H. pylori* and salmonella. Onion extract even caused a remission in a group of HIV-positive individuals. In lab studies onion extract inhibits the spread of human breast cancer, lung, colon, liver and prostate cells. Research shows that adding onion powder to hamburger before cooking can inactivate formation of carcinogens.

Of all onion's talents, the best documented is its strong anti-diabetic and blood-pressure lowering activity. In one study, patients who took a daily capsule of 162 mg of onion-derived quercetin for six weeks saw their blood pressure drop significantly. Other research shows that eating between two and 3.5 ounces of onions a day lowered fasting blood sugar in those with type 2 diabetes. Onions may also boost production of insulin levels and help prevent diabetes complications.

Active Agents: High quercetin and sulfur compounds are credited for most of onion's health benefits.

Essential Advice: *Eat onions regularly raw or mildly cooked. Red onions have slightly higher phytochemical activity than white or yellow onions.*

POMEGRANATE

Prehistoric Miracle Fruit

Small, round, and red, the pomegranate, also called "miracle fruit" has thrived around the Mediterranean, since 3500 BC. It has multiple and diverse biochemical powers to ward off premature aging and death.

Pomegranate's juice and seeds are its greatest edible prizes. The juice has 20 percent higher disease-fighting antioxidant activity than other high-ranking juices and beverages, including apple, acai, black cherry, blueberry, cranberry, concord grape, red wine and green tea. It is also rich in phytochemicals that help counteract inflammation, ulcers, high blood pressure, infections, osteoporosis, liver damage and various cancers.

Most impressive is pomegranate juice's life-extending diversity. A string of studies show it discourages obesity, hyperglycemia, and type 2 diabetes. Evidence shows it may also slow the progression of neurodegenerative diseases, age-related memory loss and Alzheimer's disease, and even help treat osteoporosis, and prevent common infections.

Especially noteworthy is pomegranate's anti-metastasis powers that are reported to help block the spread of cancers of the lung, breast, prostate, thyroid, skin, kidney, cervix, bladder, and ovaries.

Active Agents: Researchers attribute pomegranate's powers to high concentrations of polyphenols, such as ellagic acid and anthocyanins.

Essential Advice: *Consider drinking eight ounces of pomegranate juice daily or a few times weekly. Buy commercial juice without added sugar or make it by liquifying pomegranate seeds in the blender. You can eat the seeds as well.*

POTATO

Fried Foods from Hell

Over-eating white potatoes can help give you a larger waist, less favorable blood cholesterol, and raise your blood pressure. But it's very unlikely a potato excess will push you into an early grave due to chronic diseases including heart disease, stroke or cancer *if--and here's the important caveat--you eat potatoes raw, boiled, mashed, and baked, in short "unfried."*

Extensive evidence shows that eating potatoes prepared in all ways except fried do not predispose you to premature death. For example, a recent study of 50,000 Norwegian adults found no association between how often they ate boiled white potatoes and their odds of dying.

However, there is a decided higher risk of death from eating French fried potatoes, which unfortunately make up most of the potatoes consumed in the U.S., especially in restaurants.

A recent National Institutes of Health study that focused on death rates from fried potatoes was shocking. As expected, eating lots of *unfried* potatoes did not raise death probabilities. But eating *fried* potatoes, mostly as French fries, only twice a week raised the risk of death in a group of 4400 Americans during an eight-year period by *100 percent!*

In short, eating a couple of servings of French fries a week *doubled* a potato's ordinary odds to inflict death. Eating French fried potatoes three times a week boosted death chances a further 25 to 50 percent.

Active Agents: Chemical byproducts produced by frying potatoes in high temperature oils are blamed as the main villains, notably acrylamide, often detected in French fries and potato chips.

Essential Advice: *Eat white potatoes raw, boiled, baked, mashed, or scalloped. Avoid fried potatoes, especially French fries and potato chips.*

POULTRY & WHITE MEAT

Better than Dark

You are apt to end up earlier in your permanent resting place if you eat red meat instead of white meat. Researchers at London's Imperial College reported that eating three and a half ounces of red meat a day was likely to prompt a 16 percent *increase* in cardiovascular deaths. But death rates did not rise or fall from eating the same amount of white meat, including poultry.

A ten-year National Cancer Institute study showed that death odds shot up one third in men and women who ate the most red meat compared to the least. Those eating the most white meat actually saw slight decreases in their odds of death from any cause and notably from cancer.

Particularly interesting is recent evidence suggesting that eating white meat may fend off strokes. One study predicted a rise of up to 25 percent for stroke risk from eating processed meat like bacon, etc. The zinger: Eating white meat predicted as much as a 22 percent *decrease* in stroke risk.

All meat is not an equal threat. Red is apt to be deadly. White appears to be neutral or even life extending. White meat includes poultry, game birds, rabbits, and excludes all mammal flesh which is classified as red meat.

Active Agents: A prime reason white meat is much safer than meat; it lacks high heme iron thought to be red meat's death-provoking weapon.

Essential Advice: *If you eat meat, make it white meat, not red or processed.*

PROTEIN

Plant or Animal, Deadly Difference

Your longevity depends partly on whether you get your protein primarily from a steak or a cup of beans. A Harvard analysis of the diet records of 130,000 men and women over a period of 30 years showed that plant protein promotes longevity and meat protein promotes death.

In any case, Americans rarely lack protein. Meat-eaters tend to ingest excessive protein and vegetarians get plenty of protein from nuts, beans, tofu and whole grains. Even broccoli, per calorie, has more protein than steak.

Thus, the main health issue with protein is not how much to eat but whether its source is a plant or animal. Research suggests that eating a mere three percent of your calories from plant protein cuts overall death risk by 10 percent and cardiac deaths by 12 percent. Eliminating protein-rich red meat cuts overall death risk 12 percent. Better yet, research shows the chances of premature death plummet a whopping 34 percent if you replace three percent of calories of processed red meat protein with plant protein.

Protein in nuts and seeds is particularly powerful in zapping fatal cardiovascular disease. Loma Linda University researchers found that the highest meat protein eaters were 61 percent more apt to have fatal heart disease compared with only 40 percent among those eating the most protein from nuts and seeds.

Researchers warn against getting your protein quota from multi-grain high protein bars, which are typically loaded with sugar, fat and calories. You are far better off with a snack of yogurt, carrots or fruit.

Nor are *all* plant proteins life-enhancing. For example, plant-based protein foods such as white bread, refined grains, fried potatoes, sugar-sweetened beverages, sweets, and desserts can lead to death just as efficiently as animal-based diets.

Essential Advice: *For a longer life, eat far more protein derived from "health-giving" plants than from death-promoting animals.*

RICE

Go for Brown, Not White

Rice has been the defining feature of Asian diets for several thousand years. It is a staple for about half the world's population, or about three and a half billion people.

White rice, stripped of its fiber-rich hull and innate nutrients, is massively more popular, but "unrefined" whole grain brown rice is apt to keep you alive longer. However, the worldwide evidence is somewhat inconsistent.

A 2022 study of 35,000 Japanese showed that men who ate the most rice compared with the least were 22 percent less likely to die of cardiovascular disease. A similar worldwide study found that men's overall risk of death dropped 13 percent from splurging on rice. Oddly, eating rice did not lower death rates in women.

Another study came to the disturbing and odd conclusion that women in fact who ate the most rice had an eight percent *higher* risk of death!

Additionally, a study of 350,00 Asians found a surprising 55 per cent rise in risk of type 2 diabetes among men and women who ate three to four daily servings of white rice versus one to two servings a week. Typically, white rice spikes blood sugar far more rapidly than brown rice, increasing the risk of developing diabetes.

Mahshid Dehghan, PhD, at McMaster University in Ontario says eating rice is unlikely to significantly influence the risk of heart attack or stroke and that a couple of cups of any type a day is not likely to be harmful, although most experts consider brown rice superior.

Active Agents: Experts credit the high fiber in the outer coating of brown rice for making a life and death difference.

Essential Advice*: Eat brown rice as a first choice and avoid white rice if possible. You can also substitute gluten-free quinoa for rice.*

SALT & SODIUM

Thieves of Longevity

Scientists have debated the hazards of salty food for half a century. The latest major study of half a million people was published in the European Heart Journal in July 2022. Its message is unforgettable: Salt is a mighty killer, and you will live longer if you ban it from your table.

Tulane University researchers noted that always salting your food drives up the risk of premature death by 28 percent, compared to never or rarely adding salt. Salt is found to erase 2.28 years of life expectancy for men and 1.5 years for women after middle age.

Duke University researchers discovered a direct link between average sodium intake and death rates. Even when sodium intake was fairly low, the more sodium, the higher the mortality. Death odds spurted up about 12 percent for every additional 1000 milligrams increase in sodium intake.

Another large meta-analysis of 107 studies in sixty-six countries blamed 1.65 million annual deaths from heart disease and strokes on increased use of sodium, accounting for one in ten deaths. The average sodium consumption was 3.95 grams of sodium per day.

A few studies have claimed that too *little* salt might increase death rates, but they have little credibility in academic scientific circles.

Active Agents: Salt is made up of chloride and sodium; the latter is assumed to be the malicious component, triggering high blood pressure and other damage promoting death.

Essential Advice: *The American Heart Association advises cutting salt intake to 2300 milligrams daily. The average American now eats 3400 milligrams daily. Since we get 70 percent of our sodium intake from packaged and prepared foods, read food labels and choose only packaged foods low in sodium.*

SATURATED FATS

Not the Killers You Imagine

Since the 1950's, so-called "saturated" fats in dairy foods and fatty meats have been vilified as prime instigators of high blood cholesterol and our epidemic of fatal cardiovascular disease. Common advice: avoid saturated fats or slash intake to under ten percent of daily calories.

Harvard experts agree that cutting saturated fats may help fend off a heart attack, but new evidence questions how disastrous saturated fat really is. A recent 20-year Harvard study of 350,000 men and women concluded that those who ate the most saturated fat were "no more likely to have developed heart disease or had a stroke than those with the lowest saturated fat consumption."

And a major 2020 British study concluded: "We found little or no effect of reducing saturated fat on all-cause mortality or on cardiovascular mortality." Nor did reducing intake of saturated fats lessen deaths from cancer or other diseases.

However, a conflicting Harvard study of 127,000 medical professionals did find that replacing five percent of calories from saturated fat with unsaturated fats was followed by a 25 percent drop in the risk of heart disease.

When Harvard investigators looked again in 2020 at an analysis of a million people, they affirmed that saturated fats are villains, driving up death rates from all causes, including cardiovascular disease. Every five percent increase in saturated fat calories also spiked deadly cancer risk by four percent.

Essential Advice: *Even though the evidence about saturated fat appears oddly contradictory, it is smart to cut back on its main sources: cheese, beef, pork, hot dogs, butter, lard, and other fats and oils. As one Harvard researcher said: "After all, saturated fats are definitely not health foods."*

SEAWEED

Can a Million Japanese Be Wrong?

Although edible seaweed is most popular in Asia, mainly Japan, China and Korea, it is no longer exotic in Western countries. And true to its ancient reputation, it is proving to be a vigorous life force.

It is also known as kelp (the largest variety of seaweed), wakame, kombu, nori, dulse, hijiki, Irish moss, and sea lettuce. It comes in several colors: red, green, brown, purple, typically grows in coastal waters and is often sold dried.

In a current study of over a million and a half Japanese citizens, men who ate seaweed nearly every day compared with men who never ate it, were 21 percent less apt to die of cardiovascular disease and 31 percent less apt to have a fatal stroke. Women who ate seaweed daily were 30 percent less apt to die from either cardiovascular disease or stroke.

Some researchers speculate that one reason Hong Kong ranks number one in longevity and Japan ranks number two in longevity among 193 countries or territories is their uniquely regular high consumption of seaweed.

Active Agents: Researchers identify molecules called fucoidans as seaweed's secret longevity weapon that tend to stall the aging process and promote healing and tissue regeneration.

Essential Advice: *If you haven't already, give seaweed a try. Research suggests that even an ounce and a half a week could be beneficial. In excess, it can lead to an iodine overdose.*

SHELLFISH

Untrustworthy Sea Fare

Yes, they are jewels of the sea, but as longevity providers they are wannabees. You can't count on shellfish for an omega-3 longevity fix similar to that of fatty fish. Shellfish (shrimp, lobster, crab, oysters, scallops, mussels) generally contain about 25 to 50 percent of the magic secret of longevity found in fatty fish, known as omega-3 fatty acids. Only oysters among shellfish match fatty fish for large doses of omega-3s.

After oysters, the omega-3 content of shellfish diminishes drastically: per three ounces, scallops have up to 0.34 grams of omega-3; lobster, up to 0.46 grams; clams, 0.25 milligrams; Dungeness crab, 0.24 grams.

A large worldwide review of shellfish and health concluded that eating more shellfish may raise the risk of hyperuricemia and gout, but not make you more prone to type 2 diabetes. Several studies found an insignificant connection between eating shellfish and risk of cardiovascular diseases, although low intake of shrimp and crab predicted a greater risk of stroke. Shellfish had no impact on the risk of endometriosis.

One study found that high consumption of shellfish predicted a 50 percent reduction in hip fractures. Eating shellfish more than three times a week reduced the risk of thyroid cancer 30 percent but had no impact on the risk of pancreatic cancer. A possible downside: shellfish tend to absorb mercury from sea water.

Active Agents: High protein, taurine, omega-3 fats EPA and DHA.

Essential Advice: *Assuming no toxic contamination or human allergies, there's little reason, since they are low-calorie, not to eat shellfish; however, don't count on them to add significant years to your life. And mercury contamination may be a problem.*

SOYBEANS

Say Yes to Tofu, Miso, Edamame

Who eats the most soy foods? No surprise, the Japanese, who also have the longest life expectancy in the world. A typical Japanese is reported to eat 18 pounds of soybeans per year, mostly tofu and natto, which are fermented soybeans.

A string of recent studies show a powerful marriage between soybeans and longevity. For example, Japanese men who ate soy foods only one or two times a week had much higher death rates than men who ate soy every day. In China, eating soy more than four days a week cut odds of fatal heart attack five percent. Among 92,000 Japanese men and women, eating the most fermented soy foods, mainly natto and miso, predicted ten percent lower death rates compared with eating the least soy.

A survey of 23 international studies, involving 330,826 participants, revealed that the highest consumption of soy foods was associated with a 10 percent lower overall death risk, notably due to a reduction in fatal cancer. Breast cancer deaths dropped 12 percent for each five grams per day intake of soy protein.

A large-scale Chinese investigation pronounced that eating more than two ounces of soy a day decreased stroke rates.

Active Agents: Antioxidants, including isoflavones, chlorogenic acid, caffeic acid and ferulic acids.

Essential Advice: *It makes health and longevity sense to rev up your diet with soybeans at least once or twice a week.*

SUGAR

Imposes a Hefty Death Tax

Sugar causes more deaths than gun violence, estimates the *Journal of the American Medical Association*. Added to processed foods and bottled drinks, sugar promotes fatal heart disease, stroke, obesity, diabetes, fatty liver disease and high blood pressure. Most lethal is "liquid sugar" in beverages. Common sugar-rich solid foods are pastries, candies, ice cream, jams, and plain table sugar itself.

Excess sugar wrecks the cardiovascular system, warns the governmental Centers for Disease Control and Prevention. Study subjects who ate 10 percent or more but less than 25 percent of their calories from added sugar, boosted their chances of death from cardiovascular disease by one-third. Those who got 25 percent or more of their calories from "added sugar" upped their death odds by 300 percent or *tripled* their risk of death.

In 2019 Swedish investigators released a 20-year study of 28,000 persons, comparing their sugar intake with their death rates. As suspected, gluttons for sweets who ate the most sugar were 31 per cent more apt to already have died. Cardiovascular disease was the biggest killer, jumping 40 percent in response to overloads of added sugar. Not all research found simple sugars related to cancer, but five daily grams of "liquid" sugar spiked cancer deaths by 19 percent.

Essential Advice*:* Health officials suggest a daily sugar limit of six teaspoons (100 calories) per day for women and nine teaspoons (150 calories) for men. The average American now eats double and triple that—or 17 teaspoons a day.

Foods with the Most Added Sugar: *Soda/energy/ sports drinks, 42.2 percent; Grain-based desserts, 11.9 per cent; Fruit Drinks, 8.5 percent; Candy; 5.5 percent; Ready-to-eat-cereals, 4 percent. Source: CDC, National Health, and Nutrition Examination Survey.*

SUGARY-BEVERAGES

Killers on the Loose

The liquid-sugar death toll is frighteningly high. Around 184,000 people worldwide die every year from drinking sugar-sweetened beverages, reveals a 2021 international analysis. American adults drink at least one sugar-sweetened beverage every day. One 12-ounce can of regular soda delivers the equivalent of 10 teaspoons of table sugar.

The grim reality that such beverages mimic slow-onset liquid poison is revealed in a recent 20-year study of 100,000 women at the University of California. Specifically, a daily soft drink doomed the women to 33 percent higher odds of fatal cancer. Those who drank three sugary soft drinks a week, compared with one a month, *faced 57 percent higher odds of deadly pancreatic cancer.*

A new American Cancer Society study also linked sugary soft drinks to a nine percent leap in death rates from colon cancer and a 17 percent surge from kidney cancer in both men and women.

In a new Dutch analysis, for each additional sugar-sweetened or low/no- calorie beverage consumed, overall death risk shot up nine percent. Research at Roswell Park Comprehensive Cancer Center discovered that one regular sugar sweetened cola a day boosted odds of pancreatic cancer 55 percent!

Active Agents: Sugar is thought to be the deadly culprit, although obesity due to excess sugar also promotes death independently. Eating ten and a half cups of sugar at one time is the official lethal dose.

Essential Advice: *Cut down on or cut out sugar-sweetened beverages, especially deadly soft drinks. The more you drink, the greater the death threat. Eliminating sugary soft drinks predicted a 13 percent drop-in death rates, according to recent research.*

SWEET POTATO

Perfect for Centenarians

The Japanese island of Okinawa is famous for its "longevity advantage." Among its nearly two million population, it boasts 50 centenarians per 100,000 persons, which is four to five times that of other industrialized countries. The island has 40 percent less fatal cancer and 80 percent less fatal cardiovascular disease than the United States.

After age 65 an American woman can expect to live another 19.3 years, an Okinawan woman, 22.5 years, or 16 percent longer. Comparable figures for males: 16.2 years if American, 18.5 years if Okinawan.

Experts credit this extraordinary longevity mainly to the Okinawan diet, which is dominated by sweet potatoes that for the last four centuries have provided 60 percent of all calories consumed by Okinawans. Indeed, sweet potatoes are symbolic of longevity in Okinawa and other cultures. When the officially titled "oldest woman in the world," who was Spanish, died at age 114 in 2019, her longevity was credited to two daily practices: going to church and eating a sweet potato.

The low-fat, low-calorie Okinawan diet includes green and yellow vegetables, purple sweet potatoes, soybean-based foods, fruit, and scant portions of meat, similar to the traditional Japanese diet.

Active Agents: High antioxidants in the fruit and diverse vegetables dominate this well-regarded diet, predicting a longer life.

Essential Advice: *Incorporate sweet potatoes and other plant foods of the Okinawan diet into yours.*

TEA

Dispensing Longevity for 40 Centuries

Science claims that both green and black tea are longevity potions, and there is plenty of evidence to back it up. A 2020 study of 100,000 Chinese concluded that drinking green tea more than three times a week cut death odds by 15 percent, notably from cardiovascular disease. Men who drank the most green tea compared to the least were apt to live the longest.

Black tea also has sensational longevity credentials. In 2022 researchers tracked half a million British subjects who drank black tea for a decade. The stunning verdict: drinking two or more cups of black tea daily was associated with a 13 percent drop in premature death rates, versus tea abstainers, regardless of whether drinkers added milk, cream or sugar to their tea, or drank it hot or cold.

An analysis of 39 studies by doctors at Tufts University concluded that every extra daily cup of tea of any type you drink slashes death odds one and a half percent and your risk of fatal cardiovascular disease by four percent. Other research finds more dramatic benefits among the elderly. A daily cup of tea slashed their risk of dying from any cause by eight percent and by eleven percent from cardiovascular disease.

Active Agents: Tea's longevity activity is attributed mainly to antioxidant flavonoids, which are more plentiful in green tea, popular in Asia, compared with black and oolong, more popular in the United Kingdom, United States, and other Western countries.

Essential Advice: *Drink brewed green, black or oolong tea daily or at least three times a week. Some research cautions against more than five cups a day. Instant and bottled teas typically are low in antioxidant capacity and do not increase longevity significantly.*

TELOMERE FACTOR

New Secret to Immortality

So how do foods manipulate the body's complex physiology to promote longevity or death? What mechanisms actually give instructions at the cellular level to slow or accelerate life forces?

Particularly fascinating is a newly discovered DNA factor in food, humans and animals that drives processes favoring life or death, called a telomere. It is an ever-changing tiny structure on the end of your chromosomes that controls biological activity. Certain foods incite telomeres in your body to grow longer or shrink. This is a life and death matter because decidedly *longer* telomeres, predict a longer life, and shorter telomeres shout out for death to hurry up.

Scientists also know we can influence the timing of death's arrival by eating specific foods that help determine telomere length. Tests show that longer telomeres are stimulated by nuts, coffee, whole grains, antioxidants, carotenoids in orange and dark green fruits and vegetables, low saturated fat, high monounsaturated fat, (olive oil), omega-3 fish fats, Mediterranean Diet, and multi-vitamin supplements. Supplement users had five percent longer telomeres than nonusers in one test.

Dietary tactics that lead to shorter telomeres, opening the door to death earlier are more than four drinks of alcohol per day, refined flour cereals, meat, saturated fat, butter, fried food, processed meat, and sugar-sweetened beverages.

Active Agents: Longer telomeres that prolong life expectancy.

Essential Advice: *Eat foods that promote longer telomeres and avoid foods that shorten telomeres, hastening death.*

TOMATO

Packed with Lifegiving Antioxidants

No question, enthusiastic tomato eaters escape death longer. Strong evidence comes from a 2019 investigation of tomatoes and death rates in nearly 25,000 American middle-aged men and women over a six-year period. Those who ate the most tomatoes—nearly two cups a day—were 14 percent less apt to die of any cause than those eating the least—a couple of tablespoons a day.

The greater tomato consumers, in comparison, also were 24 percent less apt to die of cardiovascular disease and 30 percent less likely to have a fatal stroke or other deadly cerebrovascular disease. Moreover, research published in *the British Journal of Nutrition* found that death rates dropped as intake of an antioxidant called lycopene, which gives tomatoes their red pigment, went up.

Tomatoes also have strong anticancer activity. Eating lots of tomatoes is tied to a lower risk of cancers of the stomach, colon, rectal, breast and especially prostate, according to numerous reports. Men who ate canned and cooked tomatoes five to six times a week were 28 percent less apt to have prostate cancer than non-tomato eaters.

Active Agents: Experts agree that the main driver of the tomato's death-defying activities is lycopene, a powerful antioxidant in all tomato products, including ketchup, tomato paste, and tomato sauce.

Essential Advice: *Eat two or more cups of tomatoes a day. Cooked tomatoes provide more lycopene than raw tomatoes.*

TRIGLYCERIDES

Death Threats to the Heart

If your triglycerides, a type of fat in your blood, are high--above 200 mg/dL--you are 25 percent more apt to die of cardiovascular disease than if they are below 150 mg/dL, warns the Cleveland Clinic. Indeed, the higher your triglycerides, the more likely you are to develop atherosclerosis, which triggers inflammation, leading to widespread plaque buildup in your carotid, coronary and peripheral arteries that carry vital blood to your brain, heart and legs and arms.

Over the years, such plaque build-up in arteries can lead to a heart attack or stroke. If your blood cholesterol is also high, along with high triglycerides, your odds of cardiac catastrophe skyrocket.

The good news: you can depress high triglycerides to safer levels by modifying your diet. According to the Cleveland Clinic, four dietary culprits raise your triglycerides: alcohol, fats, refined carbohydrates, and sugars.

Essential Advice: *How to reduce triglycerides:*

Restrict foods that have these sugary ingredients listed high on their labels: sucrose, glucose, fructose, corn syrup, high-fructose corn syrup, maltose, honey, molasses.

Drink "sugar-free" sodas and other beverages.

Substitute fresh fruit for candy and most fruit juices.

Eat only whole grains and high fiber low-sugar cereals; avoid refined grains, mainly white bread.

Substitute no-sugar spreads for jelly and preserves and extra virgin olive oil for butter.

Cut out or down on fatty meats.

Eat more omega-3 fatty fish such as salmon, mackerel, and herring.

ULTRA-PROCESSED FOODS

They Kill You Young

The best way to arrive early at your grave is to eat ultra-processed foods that give rapid rise to obesity, hypertension, strokes, cancer, heart disease, dementia, depression and other bad chronic deadly diseases.

A sure sign of ultra-processed or manufactured "fast" food is a label listing multiple unfamiliar ingredients, including lots of calories, saturated fat, salt, additives, and preservatives, such as "flavor enhancers, emulsifiers, carbonating, foaming, gelling and glazing agents."

Generally, the more ingredients on the label of a food, the more reason to avoid it. Common ultra-processed foods are chips, French fries, cookies, boxed cake mixes, energy bars, sugary drinks, and frozen meals. Packaged longevity foods often have one ingredient, such as "spinach."

Without doubt ultra-processed foods are killers. A study of 44,551 French men and women concluded that eating 10 per cent more ultra-processed foods boosted premature death rates 14 percent during seven years.

A large Australian 2020 meta-analysis found that ultra-processed foods spiked overall death risk by 28 percent. Such foods also are tied to higher rates of frailty, irritable bowel syndrome, dyspepsia, and various cancers, notably breast. Ultra-processed foods also increase the risk of depression 22 percent, obesity 50 percent, and metabolic syndrome 80 percent.

Particularly alarming is a 2019 study in Brazil linking ultra-processed foods to the premature deaths of 57,000 citizens or ten percent of the population. Officials say reducing ultra-processed foods by 50 percent would save about 29,000 lives a year!

Essential Advice: *Reject ultra- processed foods, such as processed meat and sugar-laden beverages. Substitute whole fresh fruits, vegetables, nuts, legumes, fish, and packaged foods that list just one ingredient, example: spinach.*

VEGETARIAN DIET

Powerful Secret to Living Longer

Vegetarians are at least twelve percent less apt to die of any cause than nonvegetarians. However, there is no single definition of a vegetarian diet, except it must be devoid of meat.

In a famous study of 73,308 Seventh Day Adventists, vegetarians were divided into four categories; "*semi vegetarian*" (no meat or fish); "pesco *vegetarian* "(fish but no meat); "*lacto-ovo-vegetarian*, "(eggs/dairy but no fish or meat;) and *vegan*, (no eggs, diary, fish, meat). After six years, Loma Linda University researchers declared that all versions of vegetarians had lower death odds than nonvegetarians.

The death risk dropped eight percent for "semi-vegetarians," nine percent for "lacto-ovo-vegetarians ," fifteen percent for "vegans" and a whopping nineteen percent for fish-eating vegetarians, also known as "pesco vegetarians."

Another recent international analysis of 124,700 subjects concluded that vegetarians were 29 percent less likely to die of ischemic heart disease than non-vegetarians.

Active Agents: It's unclear whether the absence of meat or extensive plant food is the greater life extender. Many studies credit lower mortality risk to nuts, fruit, cereal fiber, green salads, and plant-based diets. Meat is a known killer: a mere extra ounce and a half of red meat a day can push up death risk by ten percent, according to Harvard reports.

Essential Advice: *Eat any type" vegetarian" diet and your chances of living longer go up. Include fish and they may hit the stratosphere.*

VINEGAR

Extends Life by the Spoonful

Vinegar was found in ancient urns in Egypt and mentioned on Babylonian scrolls as long ago as 5000 BC. Also called "poor man's wine" and "sour wine," vinegar is primarily made from *fermented* apple, grape and other fruit juices, as well as barley, oats, beer and rice. Most common are apple cider and red wine vinegars.

Vinegar exhibits an array of life-extending activities. It possesses antioxidant, anti-aging, antidiabetic, antimicrobial, antitumor, anti-obesity, antihypertensive, and cholesterol-lowering activity. Research shows vinegars of various types can reduce blood pressure, soften the effects of diabetes, and help prevent cardiovascular disease, the number one cause of death worldwide.

Harvard doctors report that people who put oil and vinegar on salad five or six times a week have half the risk of fatal ischemic heart disease as those who "rarely" eat oil and vinegar dressing. Primarily, vinegar dampens rises in fasting blood glucose and improves insulin sensitivity, show-casing vinegar's powerful and reliable "anti-glycemic" effect particularly among those with diabetes.

Vinegar is also strongly anti-cancer. In lab tests Japanese rice vinegar stopped human cancer cells from spreading to colon, lung, breast, bladder, and prostate cells. Moreover, drinking a couple of tablespoons of red raspberry vinegar a day for four weeks even caused weight loss. Most important, drinking apple cider vinegar in a large 2020 study, sent fasting plasma glucose and blood cholesterol diving significantly.

Essential Advice: *Don't drink vinegar straight. Dilute a teaspoon in two tablespoons of water or mix in salad dressing and with other foods. And or drink it through a straw to avoid damage to tooth enamel. Restrict vinegar if it causes stomach irritation.*

VITAMIN SUPPLEMENTS

Death Cares Little

Taking lots of vitamins and minerals is no fix for poor longevity. A large evaluation of vitamin-mineral supplements, in the *Journal of the American Medical Association*, June 2022, is unambiguous: "Vitamin and mineral supplementation was associated with little or no benefit in preventing cancer, cardiovascular disease and death…"

Minor exception: a slight drop in cancer incidence with multivitamin use. Otherwise, benefits from individual supplements were "equivocal, minimal or absent." Even vitamin E was found to "have no benefit for mortality." A recent Johns Hopkins study found "no significant effect" of vitamin B6, vitamin A, multivitamins, antioxidants, nor iron on mortality in nearly a million patients.

Worse is the prospect of *harm.* Beta carotene was linked to a 20 percent greater risk of lung cancer and 10 percent higher risk of cardiovascular deaths. Increased hip fractures were related to vitamin A, hemorrhagic stroke to vitamin E, and kidney stones to vitamin C. In another study high levels of calcium shortened life. Neither vitamin D nor vitamin E was significantly related to increased death rates. Vitamin D was one of the few beneficial supplements, reducing cancer deaths by 13 percent in one Harvard test.

Other findings suggested neither benefit nor harm. In one study 3.4 percent of participants taking a multivitamin died in a three-and-a-half-year period, compared with 3.6 percent taking a placebo. Cancer death rates were very similar between multivitamin takers and non-users, "except for a surprising small reduction in cancer incidence with multivitamin use," according to researchers.

Essential Advice: *Taking vitamin and mineral supplements for specific reasons may make sense, but don't count on them to boost your overall longevity.*

WESTERN DIET

Blueprint for Premature Death

The Western Diet, (also called the SAD or Standard American Diet) can cut your life short by a decade, science shows. It is high-fat, high -calorie, high-meat, high-sugar, high-sodium, low-fruit-and-vegetable, and is *associated with eleven million premature deaths a year!* It is also linked to a smaller hippocampus in the brain.

Here's a comparison of the "Western Diet" with the so called "Optimal Diet:" (28 grams equal one ounce.)

	Western Diet	Optimal Diet
Whole grains:	50 g	225 grams
Vegetables:	250 g	400g(5servings)
Fruits	200 g	400g(5servings)
Nuts:	none	one handful
Legumes	none	One big cup cooked
Fish	50 g	200 g

	Western Diet	**Optimal-Diet**
Egg	one egg	half an egg
Dairy	300 g	200g 1 cup of yogurt
Refined grains	150 g	50 g bread
Red meat	100 g	zero
White meat	75 g	50 g
Sugary drinks	500 g	zero
Added plant oils	25 g	25 g
Processed meat	50 g	zero

Essential Advice: *If you give up a Western diet for an optimal diet at age 20, you can expect to live an extra ten years. If you switch at age 60, you gain an extra eight years, and after 80, expect to live an extra two to four years.*

WHOLE GRAINS

Absolute Must for a Long Life

The evidence is overwhelming and indisputable: Eating whole grains is primary in warding off fatal diseases of all kinds. Harvard studies of nearly 120,000 Americans show that for each one ounce of whole grains you eat per day, your total death risk drops five percent and your risk of dying from cardiovascular disease falls nine percent.

A National Institutes of Health study of 367,442 Americans reported that as the intake of whole grains increased, death rates steadily declined as much as 19 percent. Eating three daily ounces of whole grains lowered death odds from cardiovascular disease by 21 percent and from cancers, diabetes, respiratory disease, and infections by 15 to 34 percent.

Additionally, women who ate at least two whole grains per day were one-third less likely to die from an inflammatory or infectious disease. Among half a million men and women, eating whole grains slashed the deadly risk of colon cancer by 21 percent. An analysis of 786,000 individuals revealed that eating two and a half daily ounces of whole grains cut death risk from any cause by 22 percent, including cardiovascular disease and cancer.

Active Agents: Whole grains are plant seeds that include the germ, bran and endosperm, unlike refined grains that are stripped of their natural longevity powers.

Essential Advice: *Be sure labels state "100 % whole grains" on bread, pasta, cereal, barley, bulgur, buckwheat, oatmeal, popcorn, quinoa, brown and wild rice, and all grain foods. Reject instant whole grains, which equal lethal white bread in spiking blood sugar, insulin resistance, obesity, diabetes, and death.*

WINE

A Glass or Not?

In the 1970's, wine, was popularized by French scientists as the world's most fashionable health and longevity beverage. Over 23,000 studies have been done on wine and health, with conflicting results. Research suggests wine, especially red, enhances antioxidant physiological activity by improving blood cholesterol and reducing inflammation. However, despite the widespread belief that a glass or two of wine a day is a longevity potion, actual proof of it is lacking.

A more enlightening question is how much wine can you safely drink *without damaging your longevity*? Fortunately, a definitive answer is found in a mega-analysis of 83 studies of 599,912 current drinkers published in the medical journal *Lance*t in 2018.

Increased death risk appears to kick in if you regularly drink *more* than 7.5 ounces of wine a day. That amount is not guaranteed to always shorten your life, say researchers, but neither is there convincing evidence it will do no harm and certainly not that it will extend your life. Drinking more than a daily cup of wine, or binging on wine, as well as on other alcoholic drinks, is apt to speed up death rather than slow it down.

Eighty-eight thousand Americans die every year from excessive alcohol intake.

Active Agents: Besides alcohol, the greatest pharmacologically active agent in red wine is resveratrol, an antioxidant. However, in one test the longest living individuals did not have higher tissue levels of resveratrol than those who died early.

Essential Advice: *To avoid triggering premature death, it's smart to keep wine intake under 7.5 ounces a day or less. Other option: drink wine from which the alcohol has been removed--nonalcoholic wine—or no wine at all.*

YOGURT

Gives Women a Longer Life

To find out if people who eat yogurt live longer, Harvard researchers tracked over 80,000 American women and 40,000 men for a quarter of a century, recording how much yogurt they ate and how long they lived.

Conclusion: Women who ate yogurt once to three times a month had an eleven percent *lower* risk of death than non-yogurt eaters. However, higher doses did not proportionately expand life further. Women who ate yogurt more than four times a week realized only an eight percent drop in death risk, revealing no further mortality benefits.

More disappointing, men who ate moderate to high amounts of yogurt did *not* live significantly longer than non-yogurt eaters in this large Harvard investigation.

Interestingly a large study in the Middle East found a seven percent drop-in death rates from all causes, including cardiovascular disease but not cancer, among middle-aged men and women who ate half a serving of yogurt a day. Additional international studies have reported that half a serving of yogurt daily was linked to a 14 percent reduction in cardiovascular deaths.

A most recent Harvard study documented a 16 percent drop in fatal colon cancer in women who ate the most yogurt compared to the least for 20 years prior to the cancer diagnosis.

Active Agents: Theoretically, yogurt modifies microbes in the intestinal tract leading to beneficial changes related to longevity.

Essential Advice: *It is probable that women boost longevity by eating yogurt. The evidence is unclear for men, but neither is there any suggestion of harm. The U.S. Department of Agriculture approves of one to three cups of yogurt per day for adults.*

APPENDIX BIBLIOGRAPHY

Major Sources of Research from Worldwide Scientific Journals

The author consulted hundreds of articles in leading scientific journals as source material for this book. Below are citations of major research articles used to support the information and conclusions in this book. All such scientific studies, as well as countless others on the subject, are indexed and available online through an extensive federal government library service known as pub med operated by the National Library of Medicine at the National Institutes of Health in Bethesda, Maryland. The studies are listed by title alphabetically and typically include a single first author and abbreviated publication reference.

A Prospective Study of Fruit Juice Consumption and the Risk of Overall and Cardiovascular Disease Mortality, Zhuang Zhang, Nutrients 2022 May 19;14(10)

Adding salt to foods and hazard of premature mortality. Ma H, Manson JE, Qi L., Eur Heart, et al, Aug 7, 2022 :2878-2888.

Alcohol consumption in later life and reaching longevity: the Netherlands Cohort Study, Piet A. Van den Brandt, Age and Ageing 2020; 49: 395-402.

An Evidence Base for Heart Disease Prevention Using a Mediterranean Diet Comprised Primarily of Vegetarian Food, Umesh C Gupta, Recent Adv Food Nutr Agric. 2023 Jul 25.

Association of Dietary Carrot/Carotene Intakes with Colorectal Cancer Incidence and Mortality in the Prostate, Lung, Colorectal, and Ovarian Cancer Screening Trial, Zongze Jiang, Front Nutr. 2022 Jun 17:

Association of Total Nut, Tree Nut, Peanut, and Peanut Butter Consumption with Cancer Incidence and Mortality: A Comprehensive Systematic Review and Dose-Response Meta-Analysis of Observational Studies. Naghshi S. Adv Nutr. 2021 Jun 1;12(3):793-808

Association between Wine Consumption with Cardiovascular Disease and Cardiovascular Mortality: A Systematic Review and Meta-Analysis, Maribel Luceron-Lucas-Torres, Nutrients. 2023 Jun 17;15(12):2785.

Association between dairy consumption and cardiovascular disease events, bone fracture and all-cause mortality, Jing Guo, PLoS One. 2022 Sep 9;17(9): e0271168.

Association of Low-Carbohydrate and Low-Fat Diets with Mortality Among US Adults. Shan Z, JAMA Intern Med. 2020 Apr 1;180(4):513-523.

Association Between Dietary Factors and Mortality from Heart Disease, Stroke, and Type 2 Diabetes in the United States. Micha R. JAMA. 2017 Mar 7;317(9): 55

Association between patterns of alcohol consumption (beverage type, frequency and consumption with food) and risk of adverse health outcomes: a cohort study, Bhautesh Dinesh Jani, et al, BMC Med. 2021 Jan 12;19(1):8.

Association of poultry consumption with cardiovascular diseases and all-cause mortality: a systematic review and dose response meta-analysis of prospective cohort studies. Papp RE, Crit Rev Food Sci Nutr. 2023;63(15):2366-2387.

Association of Sugar-Sweetened, Artificially Sweetened, and Unsweetened Coffee Consumption with All-Cause and Cause-Specific Mortality: A Large Prospective Cohort Study, Dan Liu, Ann Intern Med. 2022 Jul;175(7):909-917.

Association of Dietary Fiber, Composite Dietary Antioxidant Index and Risk of Death in Tumor Survivors: National Health and Nutrition Examination Survey 2001-2018, Zongbiao Tan, Ann Med. 2023 Dec;55(1):2221036.

Association of fried food consumption with all cause, cardiovascular, and cancer mortality: prospective cohort study. Sun Y, BMJ. 2019 J 10.1136/PMID: 30674467

Association of Low-Carbohydrate and Low-Fat Diets With Mortality Among US Adults. Shan Z,. JAMA Intern Med. 2020 Apr 1;180(4):513-523

Association of poultry consumption with cardiovascular diseases and all-cause mortality: a systematic review and dose response meta-analysis of prospective cohort studies. Papp RE, Crit Rev Food Sci Nutr. 2023;63(15):2366-2387.

Association of soy and fermented soy product intake with total and cause specific mortality: prospective cohort study, Ryoko Katagiri, BMJ 2020 Jan 29:368:m34.

Association of Sugar-Sweetened, Artificially Sweetened, and Unsweetened Coffee Consumption with All-Cause and Cause-Specific Mortality: A Large Prospective Cohort Study, Dan Liu, Ann Intern Med. 2022 Jul;175(7):909-917.

Associations of Adherence to the DASH Diet and the Mediterranean Diet with All-Cause Mortality in Subjects with Various Glucose Regulation States, Jun-Sing Wang, Front Nutr. 2022 Jan 27; 9:828792.

Associations of animal source foods, cardiovascular disease history, and health behaviors from the national health and nutrition examination survey: 2013-2016, Adam Eckart, Glob Epidemiol. 2023 May 18:5:100112.

Associations of Processed Meat, Unprocessed Red Meat, Poultry, or Fish Intake with Incident Cardiovascular Disease and All-Cause Mortality.Zhong VW, JAMA Intern Med. 2020 Apr 1;180(4):503-512.

Associations of sugar-sweetened, artificially sweetened and naturally sweet juices with all-cause mortality in 198, 285 UK Biobank participants: a prospective cohort study, Jana J Anderson, BMC Med. 2020 Apr 24;18(1):97.

Associations between dietary fiber intake and mortality from all causes, cardiovascular disease and cancer: a prospective study. Journal Translational Volume 20, Article number: 344 (2022)

Associations of dairy intake with risk of mortality in women and men: three prospective cohort studies, Ming Ding, BMJ 2019; Nov. 27:367.

Associations of dietary fiber intake with chronic inflammatory airway diseases and mortality in adults: a population-based study, Shanhong Lin, Front Public Health. 2023 May 26:11:1167167

Cardiovascular Disease Mortality and Cancer Incidence in Vegetarians: A Meta-Analysis and Systematic Review, Tao Huang, Ann Nutr Metab 2012;60:233-240.

Consumption of ultra-processed foods and eight-year risk of death from all causes and noncommunicable diseases in the ELSA-Brasil cohort, Fernanda Marcelina Silva, Int J Food Sci Nutr. 2023 Oct 11:1-10.

Cruciferous vegetable consumption and multiple health outcomes: an umbrella review of 41 systematic reviews and meta-analyses of 303 observational studies, Yi-Zi Li, Food Funct. 2022 Apr 20;13(8):4247-4259.

Diet, cardiovascular disease, and mortality in 80 countries, Andrew Mente, European *Heart Journal*, Volume 44, Issue 28, 21 July 2023, Pages 2560–2579.

Dietary components and risk of cardiovascular disease and all-cause mortality: a review of evidence from meta-analyses. Kwok CS, Eur J Prev Cardiol. 2019 Sep;26(13):1415-1429.

Dietary Factors and All-Cause Mortality in Individuals with Type 2 Diabetes: A Systematic Review and Meta-analysis of Prospective Observational Studies, Janett Barbaresko, Diabetes Care. 2023 Feb 1;46(2):469-477.

Dietary intake of total vegetable, fruit, cereal, soluble and insoluble fiber and risk of all-cause, cardiovascular, and cancer mortality: systematic review and dose-response meta-analysis of prospective cohort studies, Feifei Yao, Front Nutr. 2023 Oct 3:10:1153165

Dietary Patterns and All-Cause Mortality: A Systematic Review [Internet]. Boushey C, USDA Nutrition Evidence Systematic Review; 2020 Jul.PMID

Dairy Consumption and Total Cancer and Cancer-Specific Mortality: A Meta-Analysis of Prospective Cohort Studies, Shaoyue Jin,Advances in Nurtrition, Volume 13, Issue 4, July 2022, Pages 1063-1082.

Effect of eggplant (*Solanum melongena*) on the metabolic syndrome: A review. Yarmohammadi F,Iran J Basic Med Sci. 2021 Apr;24(4):42

Effect of long-term caloric restriction on DNA methylation measures of biological aging in healthy adults from the CALERIE trial, R. Waziry, Aging Nature, volume 3, pages 248–257 (2023

Effects of Flavonoids on Cardiovascular Health: A Review of Human Intervention Trials and Implications for Cerebrovascular Function, Amy Rees, Nutrients 2018, 10, 1852.

Effects of Intake of Apples, Pears, or Their Products on Cardiometabolic Risk Factors and Clinical Outcomes: A Systematic Review and Meta-Analysis. Gayer BA, Curr Dev Nutr. 2019 Oct 3;3(10

Egg and Dietary Cholesterol Intake and Risk of All-Cause, Cardiovascular, and Cancer Mortality: A Systematic Review and Dose-Response Meta-Analysis of Prospective Cohort

Studies, Manije Darooghegi Mofrad, Front Nutr. 2022 May 27:9:878979.

Evaluation of Dietary Patterns and All-Cause Mortality: A Systematic Review. English LK, JAMA Netw Open. 2021 Aug 2;4(8): e2122277.

Fish consumption and risk of prostate cancer or its mortality: an updated systematic review and dose-response meta-analysis of prospective cohort studies, Niloofar Eshaghian, Front Nutr. 2023 Aug 1:10:12211029.

Food groups and risk of all-cause mortality: a systematic review and meta-analysis of prospective studies. Schwingshackl L, Nutr. 2017 Jun;105(6):1462-1473.

Food Intake and Colorectal Cancer. Kumar A,Indian GN.Nutr Cancer. 2023;75(9):1710-1742

Fruit and Vegetable Intake and Mortality: Results From 2 Prospective Cohort Studies of US Men and Women and a Meta-Analysis of 26 Cohort Studies. Wang DD, Circulation. 2021 Apr 27;143(17):1642-1654.

Fruit and vegetable intake and the risk of cardiovascular disease, total cancer and all-cause mortality-a systematic review and dose-response meta-analysis of prospective studies. Aune D, Int J Epidemiol. 2017 Jun 1;46(3):1029-1056.

Fruit and vegetable consumption, cardiovascular disease, and all-cause mortality in China. Wang J,. Sci China Life Sci. 2022 Jan;65(1):119-128.

Fruit and vegetable consumption and mortality from all causes, cardiovascular disease, and cancer: systematic review and dose-response meta-analysis of prospective cohort studies. Wang X, BMJ. 2014 Jul 29;349: g4490.

Fruit, vegetable, and legume intake, and cardiovascular disease and deaths in 18 countries (PURE): a prospective cohort study. Miller V, Prospective Urban Rural Epidemiology (PURE) study investigators. Lancet. 2017 Nov 4;390(10107):2037-2049

Global Association between Egg Intake and the Incidence and Mortality of Ischemic Heart Disease-An Ecological Study, Norie Sugihara, Int J Environ Res Public Health. 2023 Feb 25;20(5):4138.

Health Benefits of Culinary Herbs and Spices, T. Alan Jiang, Journal of AOAC International Vol. 102, No. 2, 2019.

Healthy Eating Patterns and Risk of Total and Cause-Specific Mortality, Walter C. Willett, MD, [j]*JAMA Intern Med.* 2023;183(2):142-153

Is Butter Back? A Systematic Review and Meta-Analysis of Butter Consumption and Risk of Cardiovascular Disease, Diabetes, and Total Mortality. Pimpin L, Collection 2016.PMID: 27355649 Review.

Inverse Association of Poultry, Fish, and Plant Protein Consumption with the Incidence of Cardiovascular Disease. Chrysant SG, Cardiol Rev. 2022 Sep-Oct 01;30(5):247-252.

Longitudinal Association of Nutrition Consumption and the Risk of Cardiovascular Events: A Prospective Cohort Study in the Eastern Mediterranean Region, Noushin Mohammadifard, Front. Nutr., 21 January 2021 and Sec. Nutritional Epidemiology Volume 7 – 2020.

Marine omega-3 fatty acid supplementation and prevention of cardiovascular disease: update on the randomized trial evidence, Shari S Bassuk, et al, Cardiovasc Res. 2023 Jun 13;119(6):1297-1309.

Milk intake and risk of mortality and fractures in women and men: cohort studies, Karl Michaelsson,, BMJ 014;349:. PMID: 25352269

Moderate Consumption of Beer and Its Effects on Cardiovascular and Metabolic Health: An Updated Review of Recent Scientific Evidence, Ascension Marcos, Nutrients. 2021 Mar 9;13(3):879

Mortality attributable to diets low in fruits, vegetables, and whole grains in Brazil in 2019: evidencing regional health inequalities. Parajára MC, Public Health. 2023 Sep 27; 224:123-130.

Nut consumption and risk of cardiovascular disease, total cancer, all-cause and cause-specific mortality: a systematic review and dose-response meta-analysis of prospective studies, D Aune, BMC medicine 14 (1), 1-14, 2016

Nuts: Natural Pleiotropic Nutraceuticals. Ros E, Singh Nutrients. 2021 Sep 19;13(9):3269.

Nutrition and longevity - From mechanisms to uncertainties. Ekmekcioglu, C.Crit Rev Food Sci Nutr. 2020;60(18):3063-3082.

Pasteurized non-fermented cow's milk but not fermented milk is a promoter of aging and increased mortality, Bodo C Melnik, Ageing Res Rev. 2021 May:67:101270.

Plant-based diet and its effect on coronary artery disease: A narrative review, Priyal Mehta, World J Clin Cases. 2023 Jul 16;11(20):4752-4762.

Plant-based dietary patterns, genetic predisposition and risk of colorectal cancer: a prospective study from the UK Biobank, Fubin Liu, J Transl Med. 2023 Sep 27;21(1):

Plant Foods, Antioxidant Biomarkers, and the Risk of Cardiovascular Disease, Cancer, and Mortality: A Review of the Evidence. Aune D, Adv Nutr. 2019 Nov 1;10(Suppl_4): S404-S421

Promising Nutritional Fruits Against Cardiovascular Diseases: An Overview of Experimental Evidence and Understanding Their Mechanisms of Action. Zuraini NZA, Vasc Health Risk Manag. 2021 Nov 23; 17:739-769.

Racial and Ethnic Differences in the Association of Low-Carbohydrate Diet with Mortality in the Multi-Ethnic Study of Atherosclerosis. Seung-Won Oh, JAMA Netw Open. 2022 Oct 3;5(10): e2237552.

Ready-to-Eat Cereal Consumption with Total and Cause-Specific Mortality: Prospective Analysis of 367,442 Individuals, Min Xu, J Am Coll Nutr. 2016; 35(3):217-223.

Reassessing the Effects of Dietary Fat on Cardiovascular Disease in China: A Review of the Last Three Decades, Wei Zeng, Nutrients. 2023 Sept (19):4214.

Red meat consumption and all-cause and cardiovascular mortality: results from the UK Biobank study, M. Wang. 2022 Aug;61(5):2543-2553.

Red/Processed meat consumption and non-cancer-related outcomes in humans: umbrella review, Xingxia Zhang, Br J Nutr. 2023 Aug 14;130(3):484-494.

Replacing red and processed meat with lean or fatty fish and all-cause and cause-specific mortality in Norwegian Women. a prospective cohort study, Torill M Enget Jensen, Br J Nutr. 2023 Sep 11:1-13.

Relationship between chocolate consumption and overall and cause-specific mortality, systematic review and updated meta-analysis, Bin Zhao, Eur J Epidemiol. 2022 Apr;37(4):321-333.

Relationship between fermented food intake and mortality risk in the European Prospective Investigation into Cancer and Nutrition-Netherlands cohort, Jaike Praagman, Br J Nutr. 2015 Feb 14;113(3):498-0506.

Role of Total, Red, Processed, and White Meat Consumption in Stroke Incidence and Mortality: A Systematic Review and Meta-Analysis of Prospective Cohort Studies. Kim K, J Am Heart Assoc. 2017 Aug 30;6(9): e005983.

Simple sugar intake and cancer incidence, cancer mortality and all-cause mortality: A cohort study from the PREDIMED trial, Juan C Laguna,Clin Nutr. 2021 Oct;40(10):5269-5277.

Soy, Soy Isoflavones, and Protein Intake in Relation to Mortality from All Causes, Cancers, and Cardiovascular Diseases: A Systematic Review and Dose-Response Meta-Analysis of Prospective Cohort Studies, Seyed Mostafa Nachvak, Acad Nutr Diet. 2019 Sep;119(9):1483-1500.

White Meat Consumption, All-Cause Mortality, and Cardiovascular Events: A Meta-Analysis of Prospective Cohort Studies. Lupoli R, Nutrients. 2021 Feb 20;13(2):676.

Whole grain consumption and risk of cardiovascular disease, cancer, and all cause and cause specific mortality: systematic review and dose-response meta-analysis of prospective. D Aune, et al BMJ 353, 2016.

Yogurt consumption and colorectal cancer incidence and mortality in the Nurses' Health Study and the Health Professionals Follow-Up Study, Karin B Michels, Am J Clin Nutr. 2020 Dec 10;112(6):1566-1575

Yogurt consumption and risk of mortality from all causes, CVD, and cancer: a comprehensive systematic review and dose-response meta-analysis of cohort studies, Helda Tutunchi, Public Health Nutr. 2023 Jun;26(6):1196-1209.

About the Author

Jean Carper is an award-winning international best-selling author of 25 books, notably on nutrition and aging, including *100 Simple Things You Can Do to Prevent Alzheimer's, Food Your Miracle Medicine,* and *Stop Aging Now!* Her books have appeared on best seller lists in the New York Times, Wall Street Journal, and The Times of London, among others.

She has contributed articles to numerous publications, including the *Washington Post*, and for 14 years wrote a weekly food column for Gannett's *USA Weekend* with a circulation of 50 million readers.

Carper received an excellence in journalism award for her groundbreaking book *Stop Aging Now!* As one of CNN's first medical correspondents, she won a prestigious ACE award for her series on brain cancer. She also won the prize for best science documentary (*Monster in the Mind*) at the University of Bergen's International Film Festival in 2016.

She is a graduate of Ohio Wesleyan University and a recipient of their Distinguished Achievement Citation, honoring her as "a crusading and pioneering journalist in the field of health and nutrition."

Made in United States
Troutdale, OR
05/17/2024

19927192R00127